Chocolate Hair
Vanilla Care

A Parent's Guide to
Beginning Natural Hair Styling

RORY MULLEN

Chocolate Hair Vanilla Care: A Parent's Guide to Beginning Natural Hair Styling
Text, Photographs, and Illustrations Copyright © 2014 by Rory Mullen

San Diego, CA

ISBN-13: 978-1500666040
ISBN-10: 1500666041

Product brands and corporate names used in this text may be trademarked. These brands and names are used only for proper identification and explanation of methods without intent to infringe or violate the rights of respective holders.

www.ChocolateHairVanillaCare.com
www.RoryMullen.com

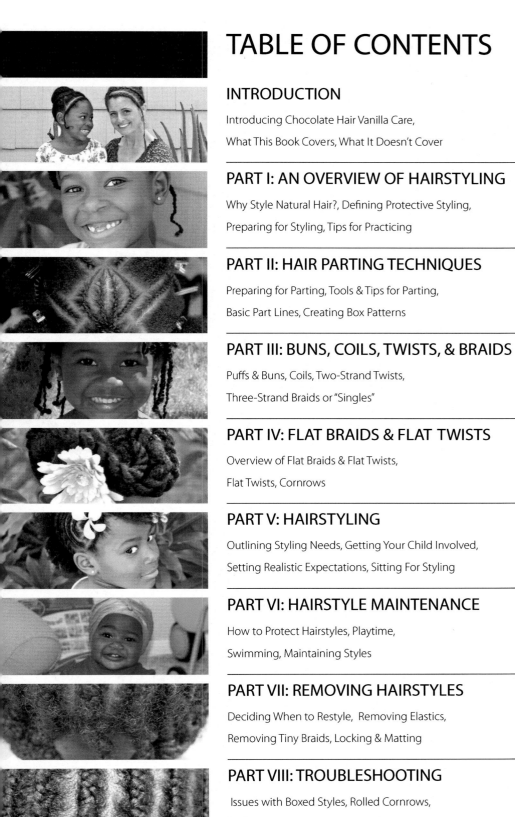

TABLE OF CONTENTS

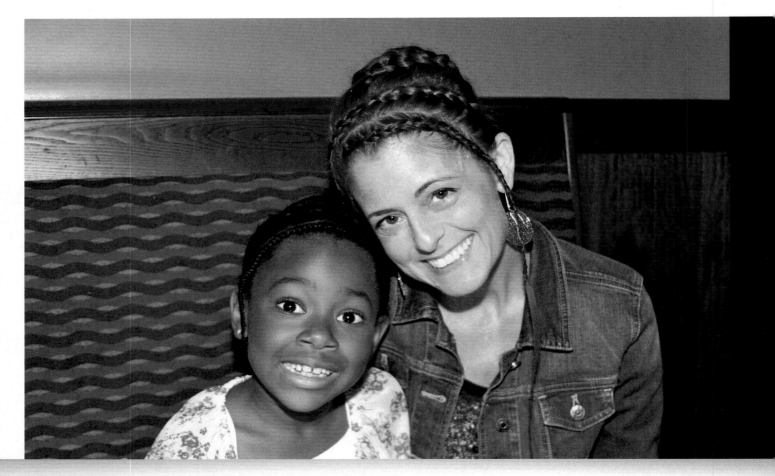

INTRODUCTION

Helmet hair and hairstyling don't really go hand-in-hand. Having ridden a motorcycle for a large portion of my adult life, the extent of my hairstyling knowledge was limited to three-strand braids—and I wasn't very good at those! Then, in 2007, my daughter joined the family through domestic adoption. After examining her full head of curls at a mere six days old, I realized her hair was clearly going to require more skills than this tomboy had.

With no formal training, I learned everything outlined herein the old-fashioned way: Through trial and error. I'm thankful to have had a friend who was a stylist advising me in the early days. However, living on the other side of the country, the bulk of her assistance came in the form of critiquing emailed photos. After the first year or so, I was plugging away on my own, trying new things, and photo journaling as a reminder to myself of what had worked and what had not. In 2010, I started posting my experiences on my blog *Chocolate Hair / Vanilla Care*. After four years of blogging and more than 150 hairstyles, I've compiled the basics of what I've learned in this book with the hope of helping others on their journey.

Evolving from my personal experience, the information and techniques outlined in these pages are by no means standards; they're merely what's worked out best for my family. A collaborative effort between me and my daughter, the hairstyles have grown both in creativity and complexity over the years.

As you read through these pages, try to remember that back in 2007 I knew *nothing* about styling hair. In short, if *I* can learn how to style natural hair, *anyone* can! Trust yourself. You can do this!

WHAT THIS BOOK COVERS

This is a hair *styling* book, not a hair *care* book. If you have reached the point where free curls no longer stay moisturized or detangled (as often happens as your child ages and the curl pattern tightens), then you are ready to approach natural hair styling. If you've been struggling to find the right product to keep your child's hair moisturized, a little bit of styling can go a long way in helping almost *any* hair product work more effectively. This book covers the basics of simple styling, teaching many of the most common techniques used for keeping naturally curly hair detangled and moisturized. Although many of the principles mentioned can be applied to both boys and girls, my experience is limited to styling my daughter's hair, which is why I use the pronoun "she" and why all of the photographs are of hairstyles for girls.

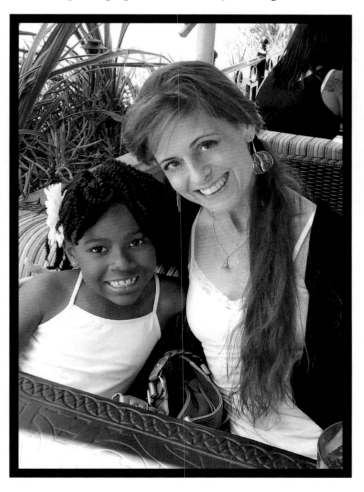

WHAT IT DOESN'T COVER

I understand that not everyone is introduced to natural hair with a newborn baby. In fact, for many, their first experience will come with older kids, be the child new to the family through adoption, foster care, the loss of a family member, or a blended relationship. Furthermore, many of these children may have had their hair chemically processed; they may have had it shaved for most of their lives; or they may be suffering from malnutrition. All of these special scenarios require hair care information outside the scope of this book. As there are plenty of hair care books on the market that cover the basics from a variety of different angles, I will assume that you already know how to keep your child's hair clean as well as how to detangle it.

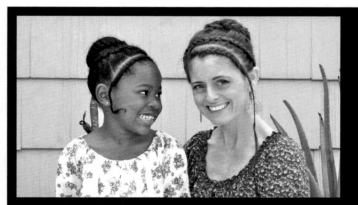

ACKNOWLEDGMENTS

Many thanks to Marissa S. Thompson, cosmetologist, fellow adoptive parent, and my first hair tutor. I'd also like to thank Michael Charles, Rebecca Elam, Timothy McKellar, Jennifer Morris, and Amber L. Wright for taking the time to read the various drafts for content and providing essential feedback. And to my amazing daughter without whom this book would not have been possible: My heartfelt gratitude for your patience, desire to serve, and compassion for others; you are my inspiration and my life.

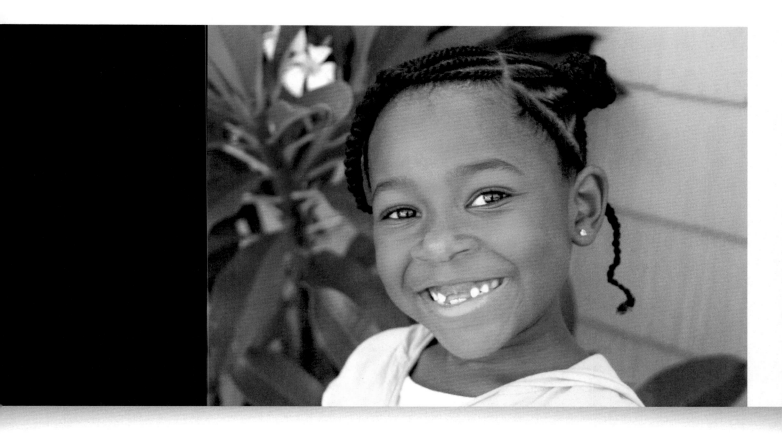

PART I
AN OVERVIEW OF HAIRSTYLING

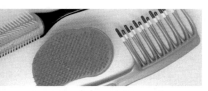

WHY STYLE NATURAL HAIR?

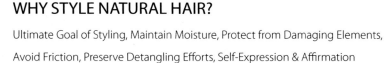

DEFINING PROTECTIVE STYLING

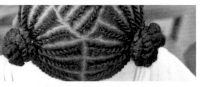

PREPARING FOR STYLING

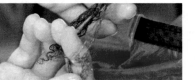

TIPS FOR PRACTICING

WHY STYLE NATURAL HAIR?

Natural curls are beautiful. They look beautiful when they're free, or even when they're gathered into little puffs. So the question is, why bother learning to style those awesome curls? The answer is simple: The longer the hair grows, or the tighter the curls become, the harder it is to keep the hair both moisturized and detangled.

Puffs are a perfectly good beginning hairstyle, especially for toddlers, because they help the child learn how to sit for styling at an early age. However, puffs do little in the way of protecting the hair as it gets longer, fills in, or changes texture as a child ages.

In short, a child's natural hair is styled to avoid breakage. Outlined on the following page are several other reasons for regularly styling those precious curls. Although many of the items apply to all types of hair, the damaging effects of moisture loss are magnified by the fragility of natural hair. Ideally, the best hairstyles for your child will help protect against breakage, thus nurturing longer and healthier hair.

Even if puffs remain a staple in your household, this book will give you options for mixing them up a bit. A simple change, such as the part lines of a hairstyle, can make a world of difference when it comes to avoiding breakage. In addition, braiding or twisting the hair in puffs can greatly reduce the amount of time spent washing and detangling.

And if you've been struggling with finding the right products to keep your child's hair moisturized, you may discover that implementing the techniques outlined in this book will help mitigate that.

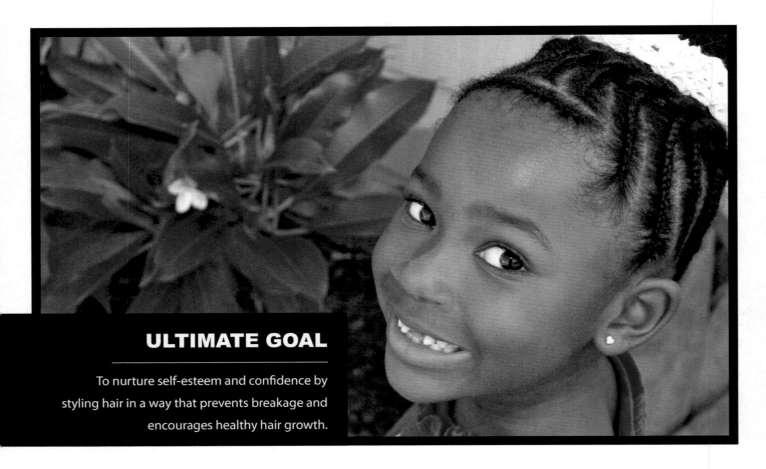

ULTIMATE GOAL

To nurture self-esteem and confidence by styling hair in a way that prevents breakage and encourages healthy hair growth.

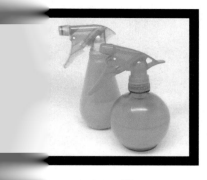

MAINTAIN MOISTURE

Moisture is the best defense against breakage because it protects the hair from other possibly damaging situations. For example, well-moisturized hair has more elasticity and will stretch into styles better without immediately snapping off. If you focus solely on one area, focus on moisture. A hairstyle that protects the hair from moisture loss, especially at the ends, promotes length retention by preventing the hair from breaking off more quickly than it grows in at the roots.

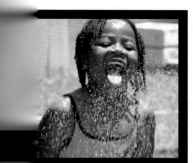

PROTECT FROM DAMAGING ELEMENTS

The sun's rays can be just as damaging to hair as they can be to skin. So can chlorine from swimming pools, salt water from the beach, dry winters, or heavy use of air conditioning or heaters. A protective hairstyle will retain moisture better under these harsh conditions. By contrast, hair that is left unstyled is exposed to the elements and runs the risk of becoming dry and brittle, which can eventually lead to breakage.

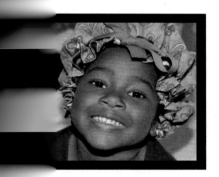

AVOID FRICTION

Any time hair rubs up against something, it runs the risk of breaking. Using sleep caps, satin pillowcases, or both are ways to combat friction between the hair and the bed while sleeping. During the day, however, wearing hair styled up off of the collar, or at the very least in a hairstyle that minimizes chafing against clothing (like jackets and collars), is yet another defense against damaging friction.

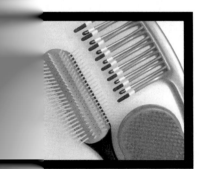

PRESERVE DETANGLING EFFORTS

Hair is most vulnerable when being manipulated, so the less you detangle your child's hair the better. However, curly hair by its very nature is tangled hair, so how do you get around that? I recommend detangling the hair once, either during or after a wash, and then styling immediately afterward to preserve your efforts and eliminate the need to detangle on a daily basis. As a bonus, styling also decreases the amount of time needed to detangle the next time around, all while keeping the hair moisturized.

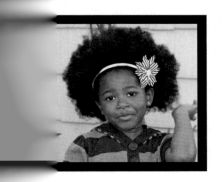

SELF-EXPRESSION & AFFIRMATION

Kids will learn to love their hair based on the behavior we model. Taking the time to do your child's hair, and to teach her how it works and why you're doing it, shows the child she's worth the effort. This is especially important for older adopted children. Learning to love the unique qualities of your child's hair will teach *her* how to love it, too. If for any reason hair care is not possible for you, please consider having someone do it who can model loving care. There's no shame in asking for help.

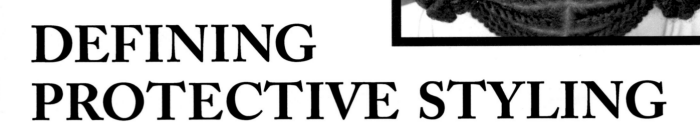

DEFINING PROTECTIVE STYLING

Whereas the previous section covered the reasons for styling natural hair, this section covers the different *types* of styles, specifically protective hairstyles. A protective hairstyle is one that helps prevent hair breakage by reducing friction and protecting the hair from the elements, all while maintaining moisture and keeping it detangled. However, not all hairstyles are created equal when it comes to minimizing breakage.

Outlined on these pages are the most common natural hair protective hairstyles. The best of these will keep the ends tucked away, though you'll notice that not all of the styles listed below do. Those that do not protect the ends require regular attention to ensure that they are being well-maintained and moisturized for the duration of the style. If you notice any breakage on the ends, then the style is not really doing its job protecting the hair.

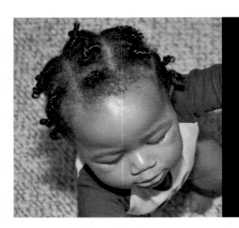

COILS

Not exactly what most consider a protective hairstyle, coils are still an excellent way to start practicing styling before your child has the length necessary for more protective techniques. They work especially well on baby hair, fine hair, or hair that is still too short to form box braids or box twists. In addition to keeping the hair detangled and moisturized, they take very little time to complete and don't require the use of elastics, which can cause breakage.

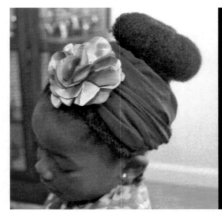

BUNS

Gathering hair into a single bun is considered a protective style *only* if the hair is shoulder length or longer; any shorter causes too much tension on the hairline. In that case, I would recommend more than one bun or an alternate hairstyle. Puffs are not typically considered a protective hairstyle because the hair coming out of the puffs is usually not protected. Elastics can cause breakage when bound too tightly or used too frequently, so use your discretion.

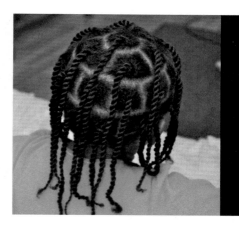

BOX BRAIDS & BOX TWISTS

When not using bands at the base, boxed hairstyles (both twists and braids) are an excellent protective style, especially when the ends are pinned up or tucked under. If the hair is long enough, they are quite versatile when it comes to styling options. To increase the longevity of boxed styles, some choose to add yarn or synthetic hair. Finishing the ends with elastics, beads, or other accessories can sometimes cause breakage, so for ultimate protection it is best to use them only as needed.

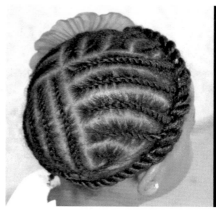

CORNROWS & FLAT TWISTS

Flat twists and flat braids (such as cornrows) are the most well-known protective styling technique. The options are limitless in terms of creativity, and they can last several weeks (or months, in some cases). However, it is important to note that flat braids and twists can be incredibly protective styles *only if not braided or twisted too tightly*. Overly tight rows can put too much stress to the scalp and, with extended usage, possibly lead to permanent hair loss due to traction alopecia.

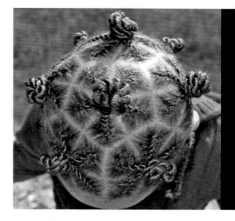

BANTU KNOTS

Although I will not be discussing Bantu knots (also known as Zulu knots, Nubian knots, or Chiney bumps), I'd like to highlight that they are an excellent protective style for those who are a bit more skilled. Formed by using twists, braids, or Ghana plaits as a base, Bantu knots are then wrapped, pinned, threaded, or just tucked into knots on the head, completely protecting the ends from moisture loss. With some clever parting skills, the possibilities are endless.

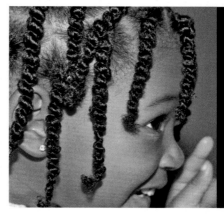

GHANA PLAITS & AFRICAN THREADING

Another more advanced technique (not covered in this book) is African hair threading, including Ghana plaits. Threading techniques keep the hair tightly bound, minimizing moisture loss while preserving detangling efforts. They can hang loosely, be threaded flat to mimic the look of flat twists, or be wrapped into Bantu knots. Gathering the loose plaits into styles using either thread or elastics increases the styling options of African threading.

PREPARING FOR STYLING

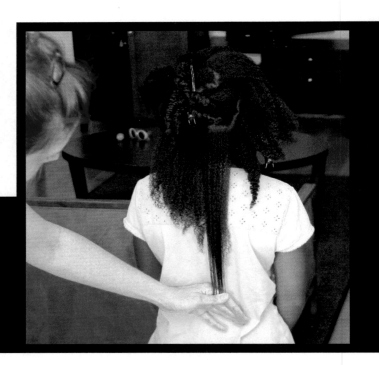

FIRST STEP IN HAIR HEALTH

Starting with freshly washed and moisturized hair will give a protective hairstyle every opportunity to do its job toward ensuring hair health.

CLEANSE

Always style clean hair. Hair is cleansed not only to remove dirt and grime, but also to wash away previous hair products. Clean hair is a blank slate onto which you can layer products for your next hairstyle. Cleanse with a sulfate-free shampoo or wash the hair with a rinse-out conditioner (*i.e.,* "co-wash," or "conditioner-only" wash), avoiding the use of baby shampoos as they are often too drying for natural hair. Make sure that no residue has built up on the scalp and that the hair and scalp are both healthy.

DETANGLE & CONDITION

Curly hair should be detangled to prevent it from matting or locking and to remove shed hairs. Always start on the ends when detangling curly hair, working your way upward toward the root. Use a combination of your fingers and, if necessary, a wide-toothed comb. Always use a leave-in conditioner/detangler, spraying with water or conditioner as needed while detangling. A good leave-in conditioner may be all that's necessary for baby hair, thin hair, or fine hair.

MOISTURIZE
(optional)

Less is more when it comes to adding products to your child's hair. Fine hair, especially baby hair, will only need the conditioning and sealing steps. Thick or coarse hair will benefit from an additional moisturizing layer, preferably with a creamy water-based moisturizer. Some moisturizing products have sealing oils in them, so to avoid build-up or weighing down your child's hair, only layer an additional sealing oil or butter if absolutely necessary.

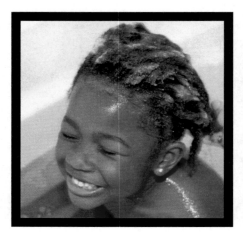

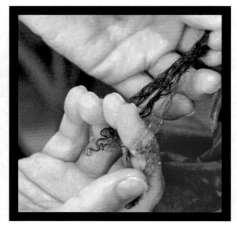

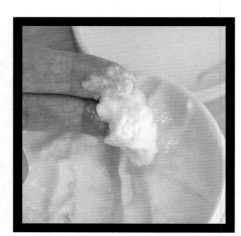

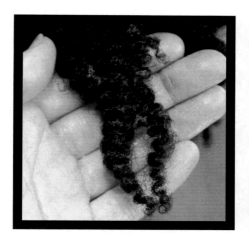

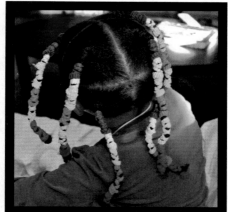

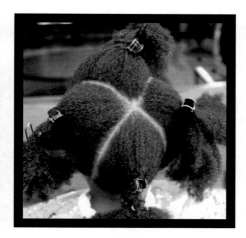

SEAL

The purpose of sealing is to help the hair retain water (*i.e.*, keep it from drying out) for the duration of the hairstyle. Since your child's hair will not be brushed or combed once you've finished styling, adding a sealing oil or butter counters the lack of oil distribution that normally occurs when brushing or combing. Sealing will lock in any conditioner and moisturizer added in the previous steps, and is necessary for *all* natural hair.

STRETCH
(optional)

Some people find it easier to work with hair that has been blow-dried straight or flat ironed because the curl pattern has been stretched. Although not the healthiest option, it can make styling easier, especially for beginners. If you do prefer to stretch the hair, try to limit it to occasional usage or for hairstyles that need it most. My preferred method of stretching is banding (pictured above), which requires no heat.

STYLE

In order to minimize fuzziness, it's best to style damp hair (*i.e.*, more dry than wet). Hair swells when it is wet and shrinks as it dries. Rather than styling tightly (which can be problematic), I've found that styling damp hair minimizes shrinkage, and thus fuzzies, without requiring added tension. This is where a good styling cream or gel would assist hold and increase the longevity of the hairstyle.

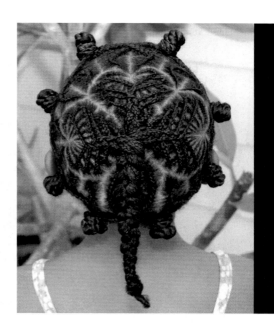

ORDER OF PREPARATION

Not everyone prepares for styling in the same way. Some people first detangle, then wash the hair in sections. Others will wash (sometimes with a style in) and then detangle. Over time, you will discover what works best for your family. There's flexibility in the order, but only to a degree. For example, sealing the hair prior to moisturizing would defeat the purpose of adding a moisturizer. In addition, you don't want to moisturize and then wash it all out, so your moisturizers would need to be added *after* cleansing. Just know that if someone's order of hair care is different than yours, it doesn't mean you're doing something wrong; it merely means that is what works best for the other person's family.

TIPS FOR PRACTICING

Everyone has his or her own method for learning, but honing skills comes with practice. Find a method that works best for you–perhaps a willing child, a friend, or even using a practice board as outlined in this section—and then *practice*.

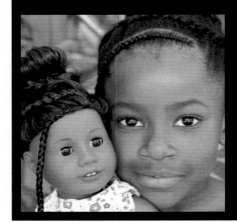 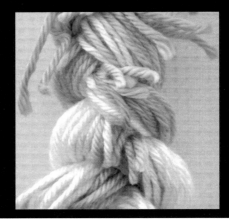 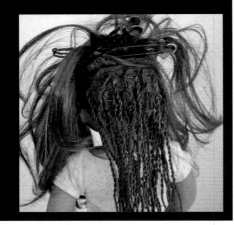

It would be great if you had friends or family on-call to teach you hands-on how to style natural hair. However, if you had someone available to teach you then you probably wouldn't be reading this book. I learned how to style hair by reading instructions, usually emails with attached photos from a friend of mine, and then practicing slowly on my daughter over the first few years of her life. If you're reading this book, you will probably be learning in a similar fashion.

If your child is a baby, you have plenty of time to practice before protective styling becomes a necessity. However, if you'd like to get a head start before your child arrives or if you want to practice for longer periods of time than your child is willing to sit, you will need another option. A volunteer who's willing to donate her time (a sibling, perhaps) would be great. If no one is available, a cosmetology mannequin head is another option. Or, to save money, you can follow my instructions on the following page for making a braiding practice board at home.

STYLING DOLL HAIR

Doll hair is certainly not the easiest hair upon which to hone your styling skills, but it did come in handy when teaching my daughter about the importance of detangling.

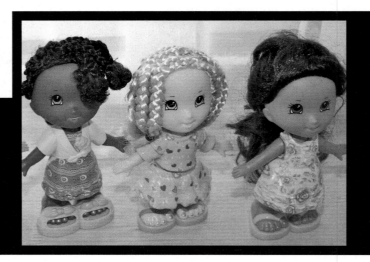

How to Create a Practice Board for Braiding & Twisting

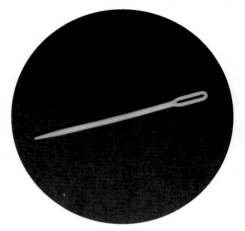

NEEDLE

You will need a darning needle (plastic or metal). Make sure the needle can fit easily through the holes of the canvas.

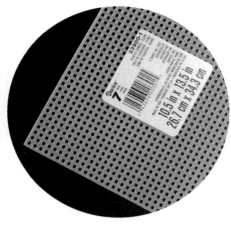

CANVAS

A plastic mesh canvas (around $1 at a craft store) is also needed. Each hole should be just large enough to slip a strand of yarn through it.

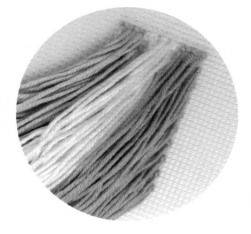

YARN

The last item you need is yarn in whatever color best matches your child's hair. I've used colored yarn for illustration purposes only.

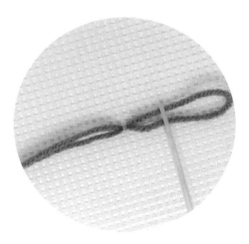

STEP 1

Take a single strand of yarn and fold it over. Then thread the folded piece through one opening on the mesh toward the bottom, then back up through the adjacent hole.

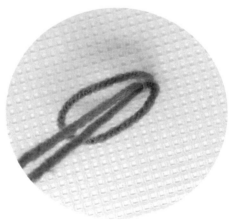

STEP 2

Take the double strands that remain on the top side of the mesh and thread them through the remaining loop, pulling taut. Repeat to fill the board with "hair."

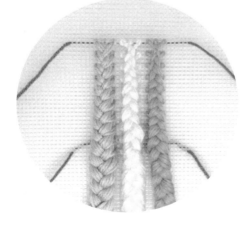

STEP 3

Using two strands of yarn, one on each side of the mesh, gently tie the mesh to the top of your leg (or any other surface) to keep it secured while practicing. You can also secure it to a table top with strong tape.

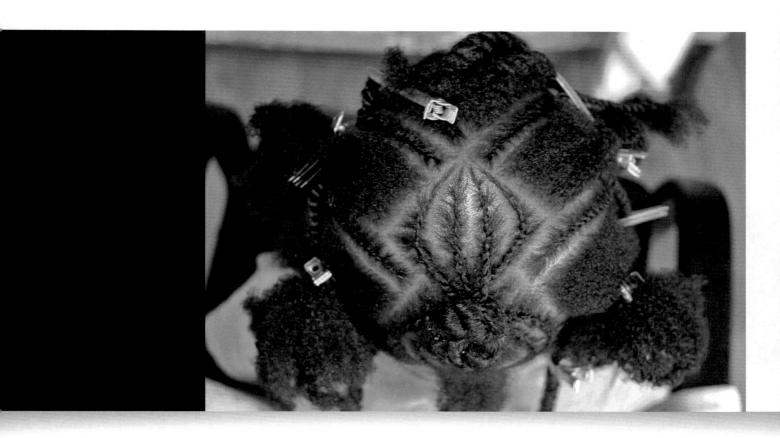

PART II
HAIR PARTING TECHNIQUES

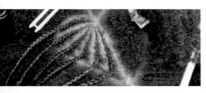

PREPARING FOR PARTING

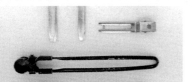

TOOLS & TIPS FOR PARTING

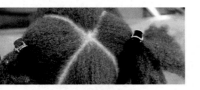

BASIC PART LINES

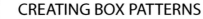

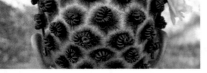

CREATING BOX PATTERNS

PREPARING FOR PARTING

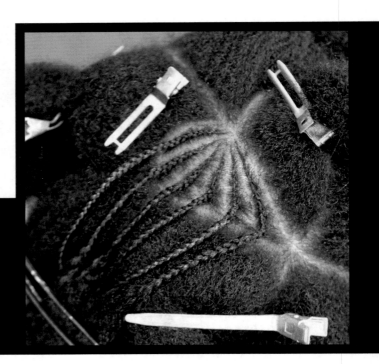

3 P's OF HAIR PARTING

If your child's hair is properly prepared, if you have a good product with a lot of "slip," and if you can summon enough patience, you can part just about any design that comes to mind.

PREPARATION

If the part line looks good to you then it's a good line. Keeping that in mind, techniques vary widely from family to family. Hair should be prepared for styling (as outlined in PART I). It also helps if the detangled hair has been plaited or twisted into sections that can be used as pre-parts (as shown below). In addition, allowing those sections to dry a bit overnight will stretch the hair, making it less likely to recoil on you when parting your lines.

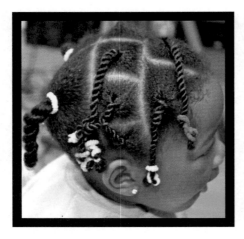

PRODUCTS

A good leave-in conditioner or sealing oil with a lot of "slip" will allow the hairs to separate easily from one another. You may choose to mix either product with distilled water in a spray bottle to spritz as needed while parting. If you're moisturizing, you may want to do so after you make your parts, especially if the moisturizer is sticky. I usually detangle and pre-part the hair with a leave-in conditioner, moisturize and seal, finish my final parts, and then add styling cream for hold.

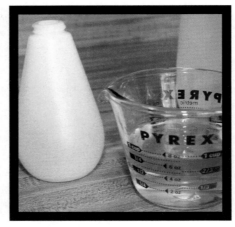

PATIENCE

Your part lines will reflect both your skill and the time invested in making them. I will very often part larger sections when plaiting the hair before bed, and then do more specific parts within those sections the following morning after the hair has had time to stretch and dry a bit. Breaking up the process gives both my daughter and I a break in styling, which minimizes frustration. In addition, we never feel rushed or like we're spending too much time doing hair.

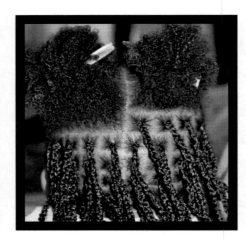

TOOLS & TIPS FOR PARTING

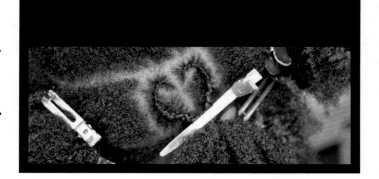

A "perfect" part is one that you can live with. If you're not braiding professionally, then the only approval you need comes from within your own home. If you like it, and your child likes it, it's a "good" part. There's no need to fuss over something that may end up causing more frustration than necessary. Be forgiving of yourself as you learn, allowing your skills a chance to develop over time. As your skill level increases you may find that your tolerance for messy parts decreases, which is perfectly normal. However, there's no need to rush the process.

TOOLS

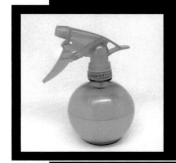

Spray Bottle

Have a spray bottle filled with a your favorite slip product (perhaps mixed with water) on standby to rehydrate if necessary.

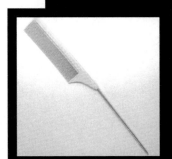

Pintail Comb

A good pintail comb will give you the fine teeth to part and separate hair, along with the metal tip to get precise lines.

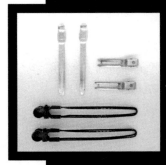

Clips

The longer the hair, and the smaller the parts, the more likely you will need a large number of clips that vary in size and strength.

TIPS

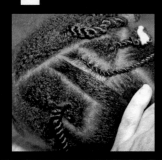

Pre-Part

Consider doing the basic parts of the style beforehand, then dividing into smaller sections as needed for the specific hairstyle.

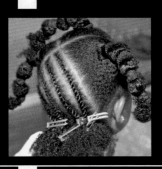

Section

Leave the hair plaited or banded in sections until you're ready to work with it, which will keep it both detangled and out of your way.

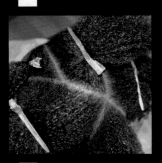

Damp Hair

Never try to separate curls when they are dry as this will likely cause breakage. I find damp hair ideal for parting.

BASIC PART LINES

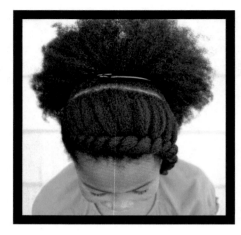
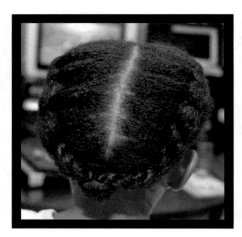
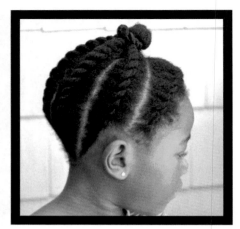

The basic part lines outlined in this section are what I use as the building blocks for all non-freeform part lines. They are essential if I'm doing anything more complicated than a single bun. I've outlined how I identify where to form the lines to section the hair in a way that can easily be translated to any child's hairline. In addition, I also show how these lines can be extrapolated into additional lines to create more complex hairstyles.

I've organized the types of part lines to flow from most basic to more free-form, complex ideas. You can approach learning them in any order, just know that some of the part lines build upon one another. Some people find it easiest to start parting rounded lines like circles and wavy sunbursts; others prefer the simplicity of starting with a single line and building off of that. The trick is finding a way that works best for you.

NOT-SO-GREAT EXPECTATIONS

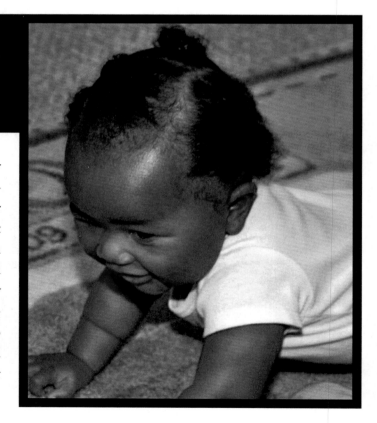

If you have a squirmy child, mastering a perfectly straight part line may be a major triumph in and of itself. This is totally normal and to be expected. Younger children in particular couldn't care less whether or not their parts are perfect. Finding the right balance between what you, as a parent, can live with and what your child can sit for is key. However, note that children will likely end up following your lead; if straight lines are important to you, as your child matures she will likely start to care more about the lines. If you have a busy family and straight parts are *not* a priority in your household, your child will likely end up not caring as much.

Front-to-Back Part Line

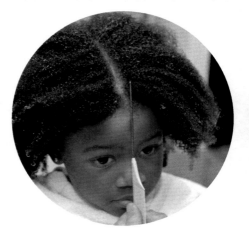

DEFINITION

The front-to-back part line divides the hair into two sections via a line from the forehead to the nape of the neck. Differences in the amount of hair on each side may vary depending on your child's hairline.

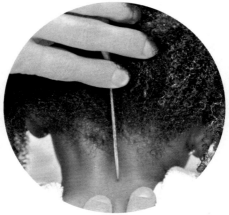

HOW

Find the center point of your child's face and separate the hair a bit at the hairline in the front. Repeat at the nape of the neck in the back. Connect the two points by gently separating the hair in a straight line.

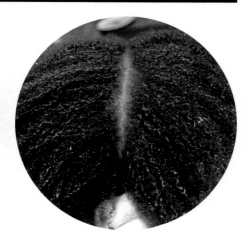

USAGE

This part line is used to form hairstyles that need an equal amount of hair on the left and right of the child's head. You can use it for puffs, braids, or as a starting point for more complicated hairstyles.

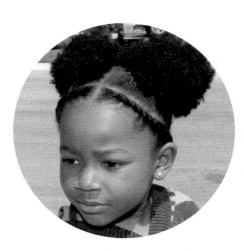

EXAMPLE

The above example shows the most typical usage of a front-to-back part line. Two puffs are formed of equal hair on both sides, along with some flat twists in the front to protect the edges of the hairline.

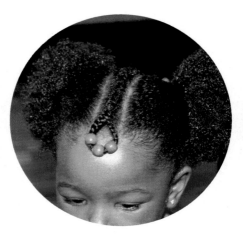

EXAMPLE

This hairstyle utilizes the center line to create a braid that divides the hair into two sections. Using a cornrow like this can help eliminate stress on the center line, which may break if parted frequently.

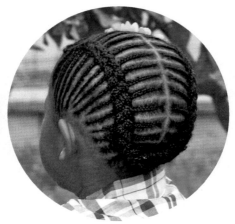

EXAMPLE

Even complicated-looking hairstyles start with the basics. The above style begins with two sections of hair parted with a front-to-back line off of which branches are parted to form the rows.

Ear-to-Ear Part Line

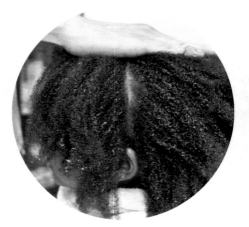

DEFINITION

The ear-to-ear part line divides the hair into two sections crossing the top of the head where the front section contains *less hair* than the back section. The line follows the same path as a headband placed behind the ears.

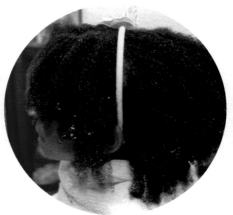

HOW

Start on one side of the head and separate a bit of hair behind the ear; repeat on the other side of the head. Then connect the two points with a straight part line crossing the top of the head.

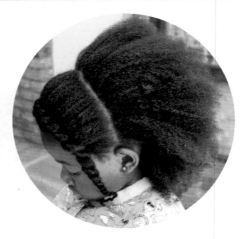

USAGE

This part line demarcates an area often used for "bangs" in hairstyles. Additionally, if your child likes to wear headbands, parting with this line keeps braids and twists out of the way of the accessory.

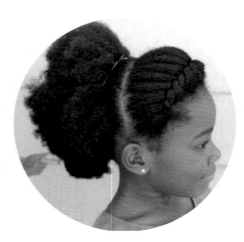

EXAMPLE

The hairstyle above illustrates how this part line is most commonly used: The front of the hair is pulled forward to create bangs, while the remaining, larger section of hair in the back is pulled into a puff.

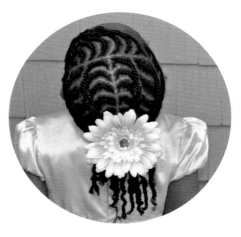

EXAMPLE

In this style, the hair in the smaller front section is braided, swooping down toward the front hairline. The larger back portion is then braided in an entirely different direction.

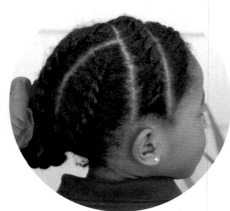

EXAMPLE

The above look illustrates how the smaller bangs section in the front can be further divided for more styling options. In fact, you can subdivide the section as many times as necessary to achieve your desired look.

Side-to-Side Part Line

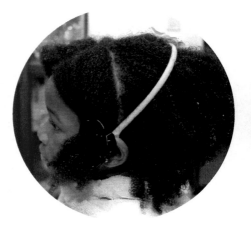

DEFINITION

The side-to-side part line also goes from one ear to the other, differing from the ear-to-ear part in that it crosses the *crown* of the head as well as divides the hair in half (so that there is an equal amount on both sides).

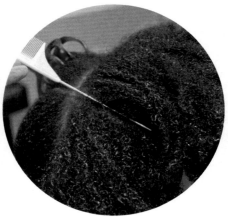

HOW

Start on one side of the head and separate a bit of hair behind the ear; repeat on the other side. Connect the two points with a straight part line crossing the crown of the head, dividing into two equal sections.

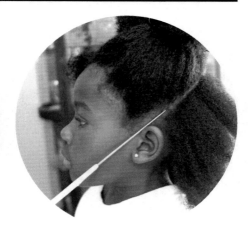

USAGE

This part line is used on its own to separate a hairstyle into a front and back look, where the front is styled one way and the back another. It is also used in conjunction with a front-to-back part to form quadrants.

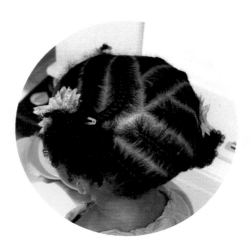

EXAMPLE

The above hairstyle shows how the front of the hair is braided in two different directions, while the back is braided into yet another direction. The front and back rows are then gathered into puffs, one on each side.

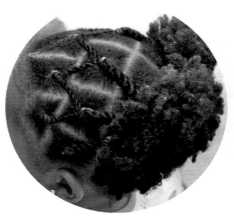

EXAMPLE

The hairstyle above is also divided into two equal sections with half the hair in the front twisted into a veil hairstyle, and the back of the hair pulled into two puffs.

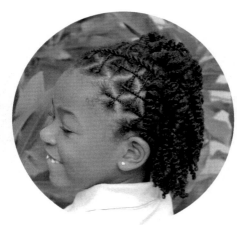

EXAMPLE

The front of this hairstyle is a piggyback veil (without elastics) that meets at the side-to-side part line. The back of the style is filled with box twists, which are ultimately styled in a twist-out to form the final look, above.

Quadrant Part Lines

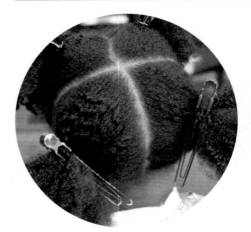

DEFINITION

Quadrant part lines are a combination of two parts that divide the hair into four equal sections, with two sections on either side of a center part line.

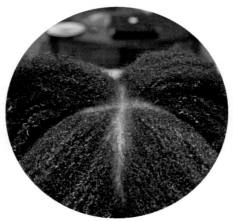

HOW

Quadrants are formed by combining a front-to-back part and a side-to-side part. Depending on your child's hairline, the boxes in the front may not be *exactly* equal with those in the back, and that's okay.

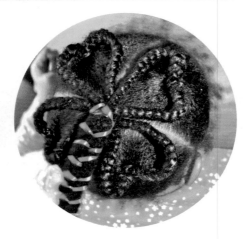

USAGE

In addition to dividing the hair into four relatively equal sections, quadrant lines pinpoint the center of the crown for hairstyles that feature a puff, bun, or other design's, such as the shamrock pictured above.

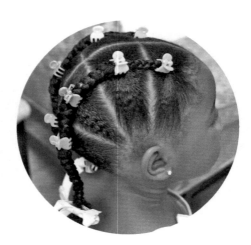

EXAMPLE

The quadrants in the hairstyle above are further divided into two additional side-to-side parts, ultimately yielding eight boxes. Four boxes on each side are then connected via two rows of piggyback braids.

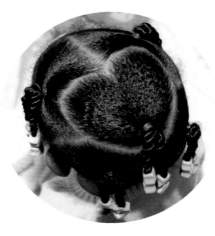

EXAMPLE

After demarcating the crown of the head with quadrant parts, a heart is parted and put into a ponytail. The remaining portions of the four quadrants are also put into ponytails, which are finished with rope twists.

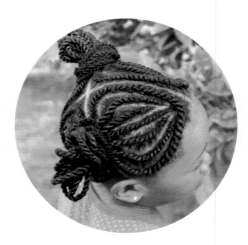

EXAMPLE

This hairstyle features all of the quadrants styled exactly the same (with flat rope twists). After finishing the designs, the tails of the two quadrants on each side are gathered into two ponytails.

X-Pattern Part Lines

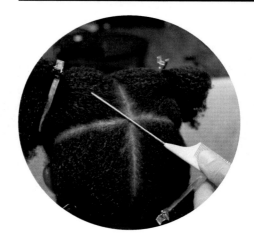

DEFINITION

Like the quadrant part lines, x-pattern parts also divide the hair into four equal sections. However, the two part lines form an x-pattern (instead of a "+" pattern) that intersects at the crown of the head.

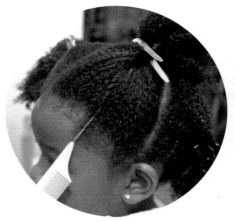

HOW

Start with quadrant part lines and use the center of each of those boxes to form the starting and ending points of your x-pattern. For example, the center of the left-front box should meet the center of the right-back box.

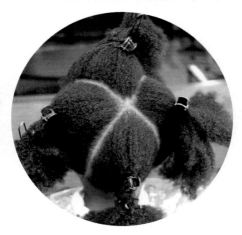

USAGE

Yielding four equal sections and identifying the crown, x-pattern parts provide a nice alternative to quadrant parts if you want four equal sections, but would like to minimize breakage by changing your part lines.

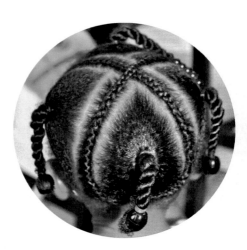

EXAMPLE

The above hairstyle uses the x-pattern as a starting point for parting a thicker "line," into which the hair is cornrowed. The remaining hair is gathered into ponytails and finished with rope twists and a single bead.

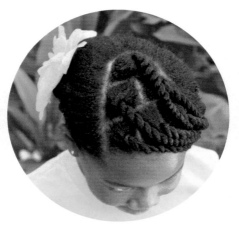

EXAMPLE

This hairstyle illustrates how you can use just a portion of the x-pattern part to form bangs in the front. The remaining hair (outside of that section) is flat twisted downward toward the hairline.

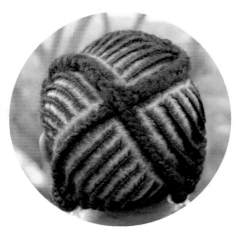

EXAMPLE

Once again, the initial x-pattern forms the center of two outer part lines, which are braided into cornrows. The remaining hair is cornrowed toward the hairline, in order to minimize breakage.

Circular Part Lines

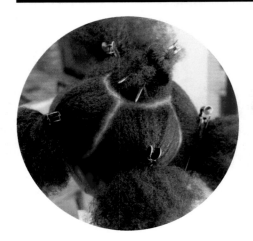

DEFINITION

Circular part lines are those that divide the hair in a circle or spiral pattern. They can be placed anywhere on the head as a single circle, multiple circles, or single or multiple spirals.

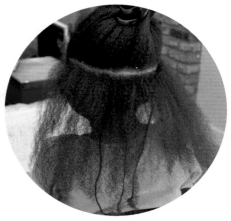

HOW

The key to achieving a nice circular part line is symmetry. You can use a template (like a paper plate) to part, but you will need to take into account your child's hairline and adjust accordingly.

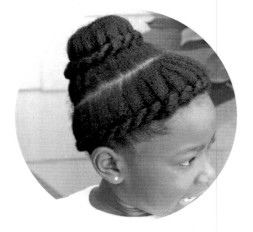

USAGE

These parts are frequently used in styles such as halos, which follow the hairline, or to outline or highlight buns and puffs. Note that circular parts are not limited to any single point of origin (*e.g.*, the crown).

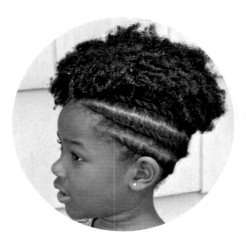

EXAMPLE

This hairstyle is formed of three semi-circles that start on the upper left-hand side of the head and move away from the front hairline and downward, around the head toward the right-hand side, leaving the top free.

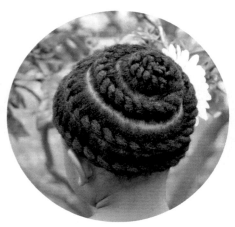

EXAMPLE

After making a quadrant part line, a spiral is parted from the crown of the head. The part now spirals toward the hairline and is then flat twisted from the hairline up toward the crown.

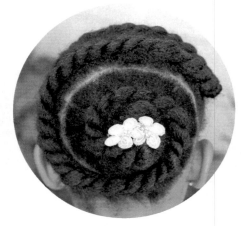

EXAMPLE

The above hairstyle illustrates how circles and spirals can be started anywhere on the head. This one is parted at the back of the head and spirals outward, then reverses direction toward the front.

Sunburst Part Lines

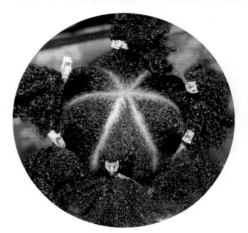

DEFINITION

Sunburst part lines divide the hair into sections where all of the part lines share a single point of origin. Sunbursts can cover the entire head or just a section. They do not need to be straight lines.

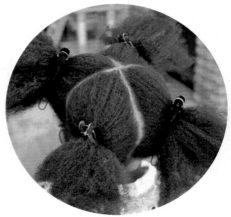

HOW

Sunbursts do not need to be formed with any of the parts explained previously. Your single point of origin, and multiple part lines moving away from that point, can cover the whole head or be limited to a section.

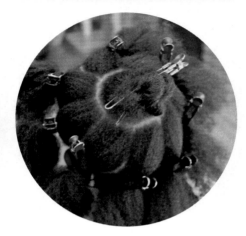

USAGE

Sunbursts are often used for designs leading up to a bun or puff at the crown of the head, or away from the crown down toward the hairline. They can also be used to create bangs or to "fill" shapes and patterns.

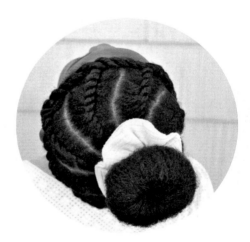

EXAMPLE

Sunbursts don't have to be centered or created with straight lines. This sunburst radiates outward from an off-center bun, with swooping parts that are flat twisted down toward the hairline, forming a halo flat twist.

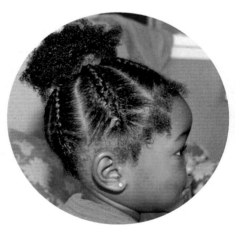

EXAMPLE

One of the most common uses of sunbursts is to form "rays" leading up to a bun or puff. This hairstyle combines quadrant and x-pattern parts, yielding 8 rows for the rays, which are cornrowed up toward the crown.

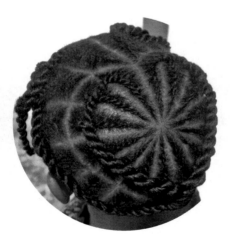

EXAMPLE

This hairstyle most clearly illustrates how sunburst parts can be used to fill in the area inside of a shape. The heart is shaped by gathering the ends of the rays in a flat rope twist to form the outline.

CREATING BOX PATTERNS

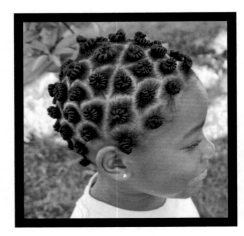 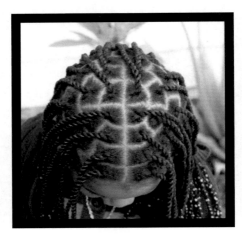 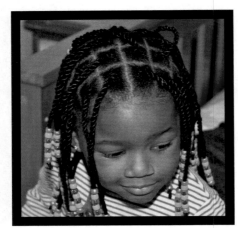

In the following pages, you will notice that many of the box patterns start with simple parts, much like the ones outlined in the previous section. If you're learning a new technique, fewer boxes are always easier until you understand how the boxes are formed; then consider increasing the number the next time you give them a try. Variables such as technique, curl pattern, weather, and activity of your child will all play a role in the visibility and crispness of a box pattern. You will eventually figure out which ones work best for you.

THINGS TO CONSIDER WHEN SELECTING A BOX PART PATTERN

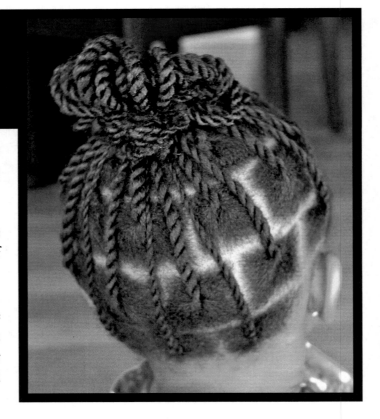

Do you want to see the part lines, or hide them? If you're not a fan of your own part lines, choose parts that are more forgiving, such as pinch part boxes or organic boxes.

How much time do you have? Some parts take more time than others and require much more precision. If you don't have the time, stick with simpler parts.

Do you plan on styling the hair after the boxes are created? If you are going to pin up twists or braids in a way that covers the part lines (*e.g.,* into small buns or rosettes), you probably don't want to invest time and effort in perfecting part lines that no one will ever see.

Pinch Part Boxes

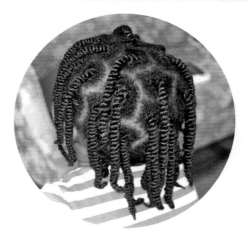

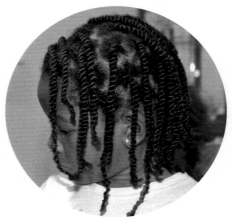

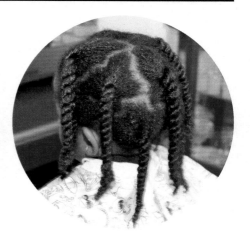

DEFINITION

Pinch parts are exactly as they sound: The "boxes" of your braids, coils, or twists are formed from sections of hair that you pinched off with your fingers. There is no right or wrong way to create these boxes.

HOW

Simply pinch a section of hair, making sure that all the shorter hairs make their way into the box. For evenly styled braids, twists, or coils, try to pinch off the same amount of hair each time.

USAGE

Pinch parts can be used for more than just hairstyles. I often use them after a wash and detangle when I'm banding or plaiting the hair to keep it sectioned before styling the following day.

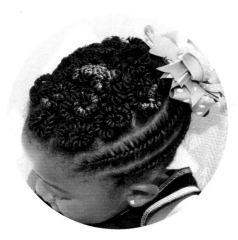

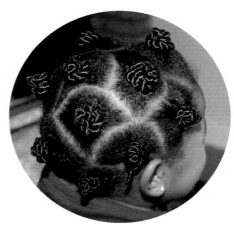

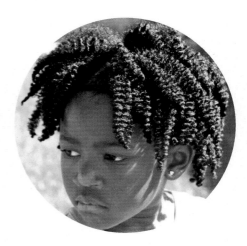

EXAMPLE

Pinch parts form the base of the twisted buns on the top of this hairstyle. Notice that you cannot see the part lines because they're covered by the buns. Pinch parts are perfect for styles with hidden part lines.

EXAMPLE

Pinch parts are a great way to form starter parts for a hairstyle where the part lines will be more visible. Start with pinch parts, then give them more definition by going over them again with a pintail comb.

EXAMPLE

Because the boxes are not uniformly created or symmetrical, pinch parts give a more natural look to a twist-out or braid-out, especially when the hair isn't particularly long or thick.

Organic Boxes

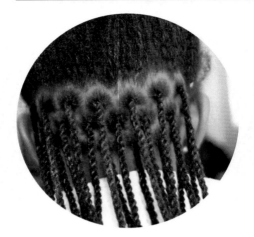

DEFINITION

Think of organic boxes as "pinch parts with a purpose." Though the overall appearance of these boxes looks symmetrical, there is much room for variations in size and shape between the boxes.

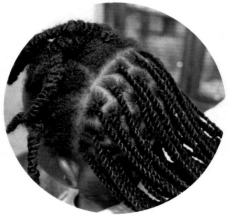

HOW

These boxes are created by parting half-moon shapes along the hairline, staggering them as you move upward toward the crown. Eyeballing the arc of your rounded edges is fine; they need not be symmetrical.

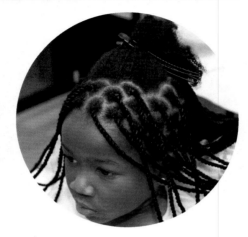

USAGE

I like to divide the hair with an ear-to-ear or side-to-side part line so that all of my boxes along the hairline look rounded and organic. Once you reach the top, some boxes may differ in shape, but that's okay.

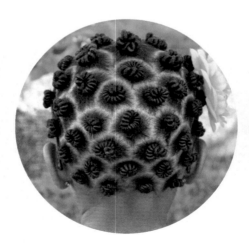

EXAMPLE

The above hairstyle perfectly exemplifies the organic boxes. Notice that the boxes are not exactly the same size or shape, but overall they work together to create a cohesive whole.

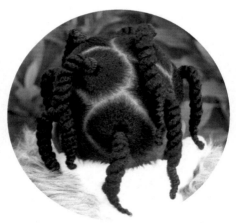

EXAMPLE

Organic boxes can be any size; they don't have to be limited to tiny spaces. Parting larger boxes, like the style above, yields a more intentional look, especially when forming chunky braids or twists.

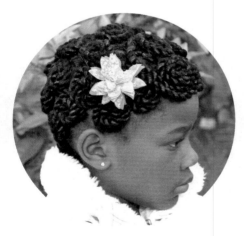

EXAMPLE

Organic parting is almost as quick as pinch parting, making it another great option for covering your part lines with mini buns or rosettes. In fact, the curves of organic parts form a great base for these styles.

Symmetrical Boxes

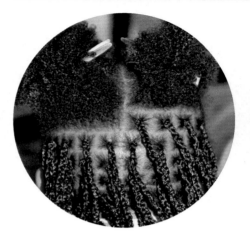

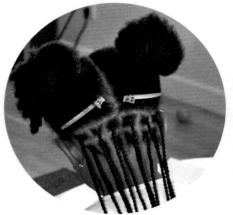

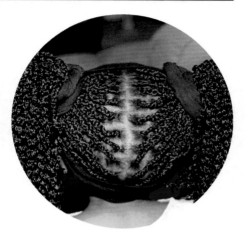

DEFINITION

Symmetrical boxes are some of the most precise boxes you can make, but they are also some of the most difficult. Straight lines are essential, which is not easy when working on a curved head.

HOW

Start these boxes with a front-to-back part line, followed by either an ear-to-ear or side-to-side part. Continue parting boxes of both equal size and number in each quadrant, aligning the boxes one on top of the other.

USAGE

Symmetrical boxes are ideal for styles that you plan to gather into ponytails. The center part line works great for two ponytails, whereas an ear-to-ear part line is perfect for gathering just the front hair into ponytails.

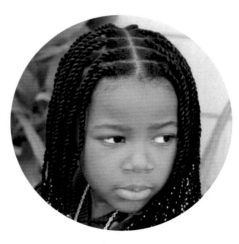

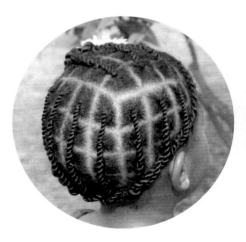

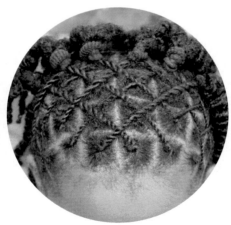

EXAMPLE

Symmetrical boxes give you a clean center part line for box braids and twists—allowing the hair to either hang evenly on both sides, or to be gathered into an equal number of ponytails on each side of the head.

EXAMPLE

In the above photo, the boxes are prominently featured as part of the hairstyle. They are connected via piggyback rope twists, styled toward the hairline, and finished with the ends twisted into a halo.

EXAMPLE

Separated into two sections via a side-to-side part, the front symmetrical boxes are rope twisted into a piggyback veil, while the back boxes form twists that are styled into a twist-out.

Brick Pattern Boxes

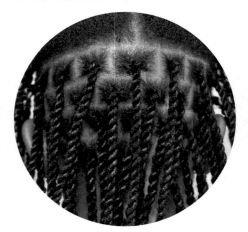

DEFINITION

Brick-pattern boxes are similar to symmetrical boxes with one exception: Each row of boxes is staggered so that the vertical "seams" between the boxes run into the *middle* of the boxes above and below. *No seams line up.*

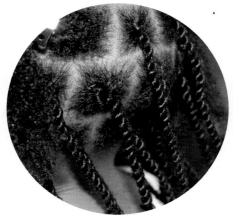

HOW

This pattern usually starts at the nape of the neck and moves up toward the crown. Start by creating a row of boxes. Then part a single box over the center seam of the first row. Continue parting boxes over the seams.

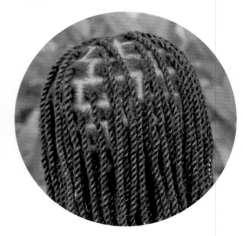

USAGE

Brick patterns are very often, but not exclusively, used to cover the part lines of the boxes below each row. Staggering the boxes allows for hanging braids and twists to lay in the gaps between the boxes of lower layers.

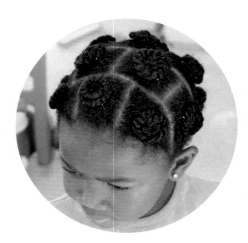

EXAMPLE

Although staggered boxes are a great way to hide the part lines of some hairstyles, they can also be used to add visual interest to clearly defined boxes, as with the pinned buns in the hairstyle above.

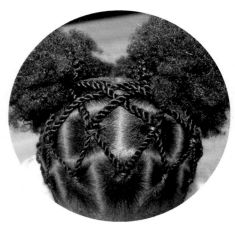

EXAMPLE

The brick pattern also lends itself to excellent veil styles. The hairstyle above once again illustrates that boxes don't need to cover the entire head. Two puffs in the back complete this look.

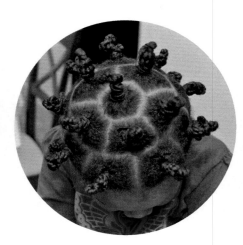

EXAMPLE

Brick patterns are a great way to work with the circular shape of your child's head. As with the above hairstyle, the brick pattern allows you to drop boxes in your rows so that you can taper them to a center point.

Triangular Boxes

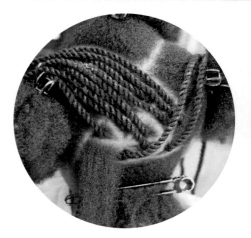

DEFINITION

Triangles can be made in a variety of shapes and sizes, using one of two methods. Good triangle parts have a clearly discernible shape; how you achieve triangular lines, however, is up to you.

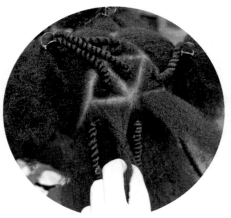

HOW

Start with an x-pattern part and work one quadrant at a time. Create a triangular box off of the center point. On each subsequent row, increase the number of triangles by two, alternating the directions of the triangles.

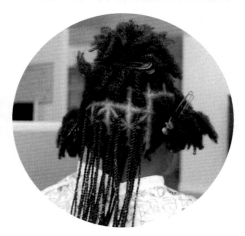

ALTERNATE

The second method requires a base of symmetrical boxes, which are then separated into two triangles via diagonal part lines. This method is slightly more complicated.

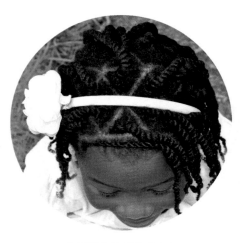

EXAMPLE

The hairstyle above illustrates how to use the first method of parting triangles for a box twist hairstyle. A flat rope twist along the front hairline gives the row of triangles above it a straight edge.

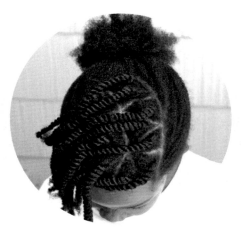

EXAMPLE

Starting with an x-pattern part, triangles are parted into just the front quadrant of the hair and used as bangs, while the remaining hair is pulled into a puff in the back.

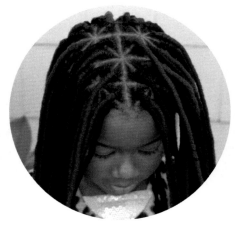

EXAMPLE

This hairstyle features the alternate technique of parting triangles by dividing boxes diagonally in half. These are yarn locs (also known as faux locs or genie locs), which are an advanced hairstyling technique.

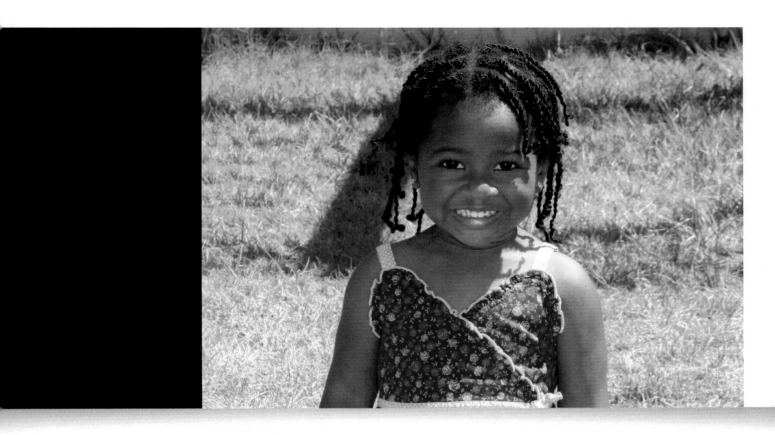

PART III
BUNS, COILS, TWISTS, & BRAIDS

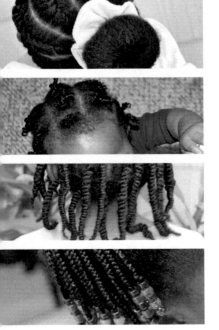

PUFFS & BUNS

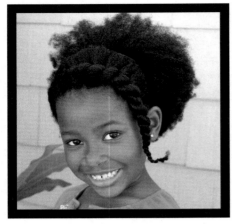 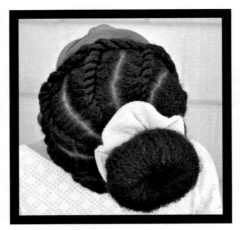 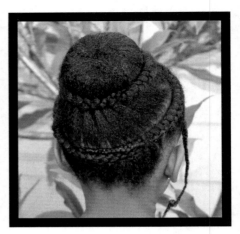

Puffs are not considered protective hairstyles because they leave the ends exposed to friction and moisture loss. Additionally, in younger children they're sometimes difficult to keep detangled if left in for any extended period of time. As a healthy alternative, I like buns. Ideally the hair should be at least shoulder length before pulling it into a single bun or puff. In addition, there needs to be enough hair in the ponytail from which a bun can be formed. If the hair is not long enough for a single bun,

consider doing a hairstyle with more than one.

The downside to puffs and buns is the tension placed on the hairline (*i.e.,* the "edges"). It's good to de-emphasize "smoothness" of the hair pulled into the bun in favor of hair health. Too much tension can cause breakage, so finding the balance between tension and protection is key. To help minimize breakage, check the market for healthy alternatives to elastics; there are several claws and clips that do a pretty good job of securing the ponytail.

How to Make a Hair Donut

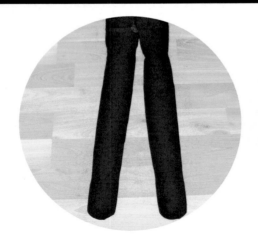 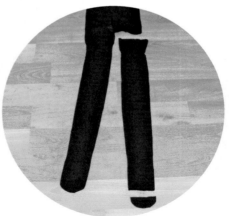 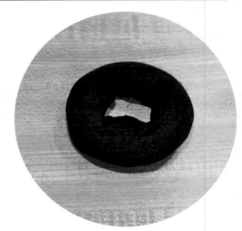

STEP 1

You will need one pair of tights or pantyhose, preferably in a color that closely matches your child's hair.

STEP 2

Starting at the top of the leg on one side, cut the leg off. Then cut off the section for the toes, which will give you a long tube.

STEP 3

Roll that tube up into a little donut that will be used for the bun. If you want a thicker donut, roll up both legs of the tights into a single bun.

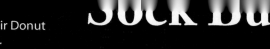
Sock Bun

- Leave-in Conditioner
- Moisturizer (for thick/coarse hair)
- Sealing Oil or Butter
- Styling Gel or Cream (optional)

- Sock Bun or Hair Donut
- Ponytail Holder
- Terrycloth Pony O
- Scarf (optional)

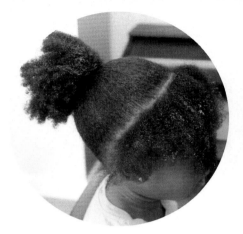

STEP 1

After detangling with a leave-in conditioner, moisturizing (if necessary, usually only for older children or those with thick/coarse hair), and sealing, gather the damp hair into a ponytail.

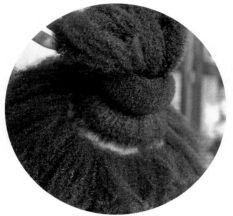

STEP 2

Slip the donut or sock bun over the ponytail. If not completed in the previous step, address any moisture needs of the hair that will form the bun.

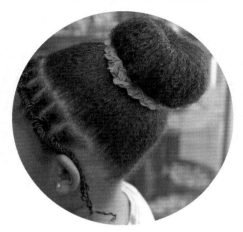

STEP 3

Using your hands, smooth the hair in the ponytail down over the sock bun, making sure it is flush with the bun. Secure the ends with a loose elastic like a scrunchie (pictured above) or terrycloth pony O.

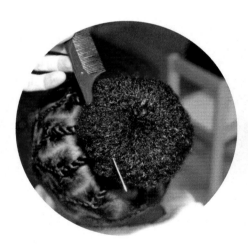

STEP 4

If you would like a fuller look, use the end of a pintail comb to fluff the hair up on the top of the bun. This will also help hide the ends of longer hair at the base of the bun.

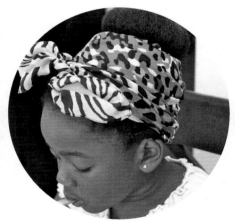

OPTIONAL

If the hair pulled into the ponytail was not styled, you can achieve a smooth look by adding gel or styling cream to the flattened hair and securing a scarf to hold the hairs in place while the product sets.

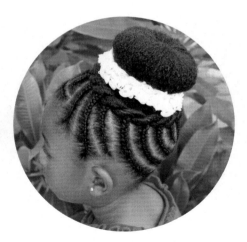

FINISHED

If either the bun or the hairs pulled into the ponytail get fuzzy during the style, refresh by repeating the steps above. Try to avoid re-combing the hair into the original ponytail to minimize manipulation and breakage.

COILS

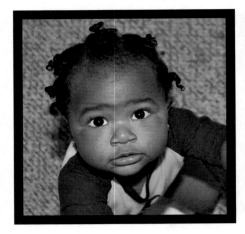
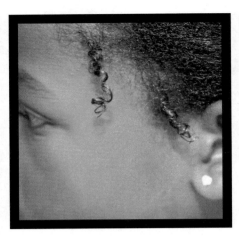
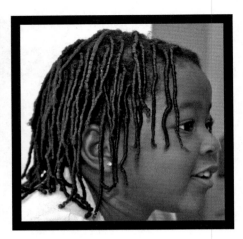

Coils are formed by wrapping a single section of hair around itself from root to tip. They can be coiled around either your finger to create finger coils, or around a comb for comb coils. Although coils are not usually considered a protective hairstyle, they are an excellent choice for promoting hair growth in babies or younger children whose hair is too short to braid or twist. They work well in both fine and coarse hair, but hold their shape better in hair that is more tightly coiled. Coils are easy to do and work equally as well for boys and girls.

Once the hair achieves a certain length, the benefits of doing braids or twists will likely outweigh the ease of doing coils. Even so, coils can still be used around the edges of the hairline, easing the tension on new hair growth while still keeping it nicely moisturized. Coils are also a good option for finishing braids or twists.

FINGER COILS VERSUS COMB COILS

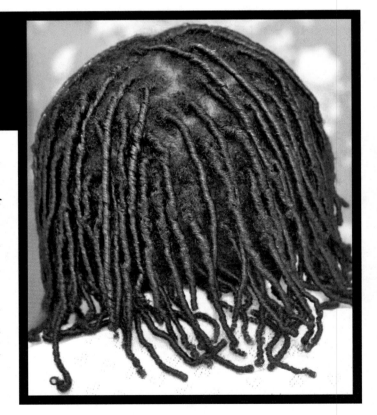

Coils can be formed in one of two ways: Either by using your fingers to twirl them into shape or by using a comb to create a more uniformly defined coil. If your child is a baby or toddler (or has otherwise had little experience sitting to have her hair styled), finger coils would likely be a good place to start. Pinch parts and some quick finger coils will give you the chance to work with your child's hair while simultaneously building trust between you and your little one. Comb coils require a bit of finesse, so I don't recommend them until you and your child have built a solid styling routine, and you feel confident enough in your skills to try them.

PRODUCTS

- Leave-in Conditioner
- Moisturizer (for thick/coarse hair)
- Sealing Oil or Butter
- Styling Gel or Cream

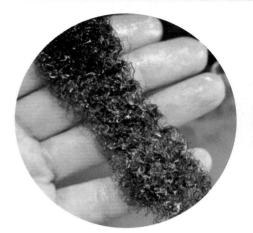

STEP 1

Start with hair that is detangled, moisturized, and sealed, and that is still reasonably damp, but not sopping wet. You will add gel or styling cream one coil at a time to achieve this look.

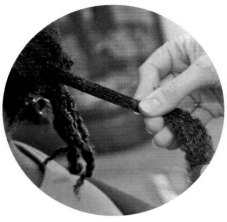

STEP 2

Take the desired section that you want to coil and run the styling cream or gel through that section, working from root to tip, smoothing the hair as you move downward.

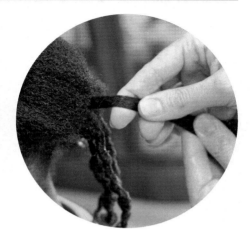

STEP 3

Beginning at the top of the section of hair, gently pull the hair taut. You will be holding the sectioned hair taut with one hand and twirling the coil with the other.

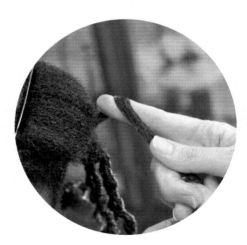

STEP 4

While holding the hair with one hand to keep it taut, start winding it around your index finger on the opposite hand.

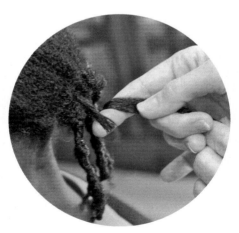

STEP 5

Continue winding the hair around your finger, letting loose the upper section when it starts to coil, working your way down toward the end of the section.

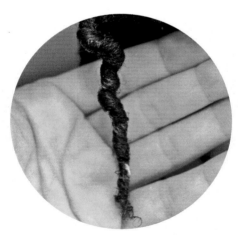

FINISHED

For finer hair, or baby hair, do not expect much from these coils. If your child naps frequently, the coils likely won't last more than a day or two. This is normal so don't worry if you don't get a lot of wear out of them.

Comb Coils

- Leave-in Conditioner
- Moisturizer (for thick/coarse hair)
- Sealing Oil or Butter
- Styling Gel or Cream

- Fine-toothed comb

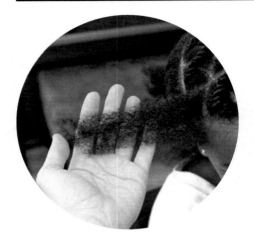

STEP 1

Start with hair that is detangled, moisturized, and sealed, and still reasonably damp, but not sopping wet. You will add gel or styling cream one coil at a time to achieve this look.

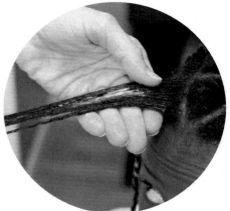

STEP 2

Take the desired section that you want to coil and run the styling cream or gel through that section. Work from root to tip, smoothing the hair down while ensuring the section remains fully detangled.

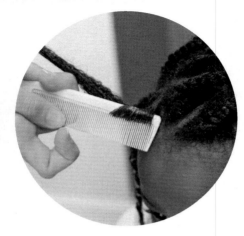

STEP 3

Starting at the root of the section of hair, gently place the hair into the upper teeth of the fine tooth comb. For longer hair, be sure to keep the rest of the section away from the teeth to keep it from getting tangled.

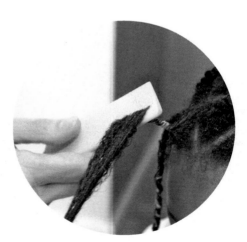

STEP 4

Holding the length of the hair section taut with one hand, flip the comb over and gently slide it downward through the section of hair.

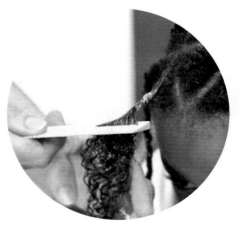

STEP 5

Keep twisting the comb through the hair, until all of the hair has been twisted. Because the comb is run through the entire section of hair, it is imperative that the section be fully detangled prior to coiling.

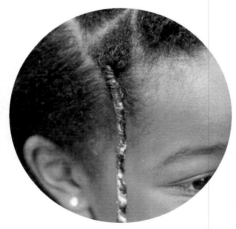

FINISHED

You will likely see hair product in the finished comb coil, which will fade as the hair dries. Also note that as the coil dries it will shrink, leaving the dried coils both shorter and narrower.

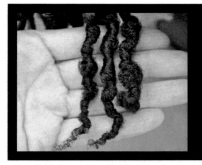

FINGER or COMB Coils?

Finger coils are usually more chunky in appearance and have a less uniform shape. They are quicker to create but don't last as long as comb coils.

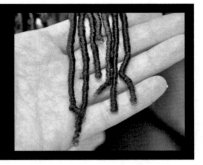

When **FINGER** Coils May Be Preferable

- When your child is sleeping or napping frequently, and a style will likely not last too long.
- When you want a hairstyle that can be done quickly.
- When you want to practice the coiling technique used for creating rope twists.
- When you want thicker coils.
- When you are not using part lines or you don't care if the part lines are hidden by the coils.

When **COMB** Coils May Be Preferable

- When your child is better able to sit for styling.
- When you feel confident in your regular coiling abilities and want to try something new.
- When you want to start locs on hair that is coarse or tightly coiled.
- When you want thinner coils.
- When you want the coils to be uniform in shape.
- When it is important to see the pattern of the boxes that you parted.

COIL STYLES

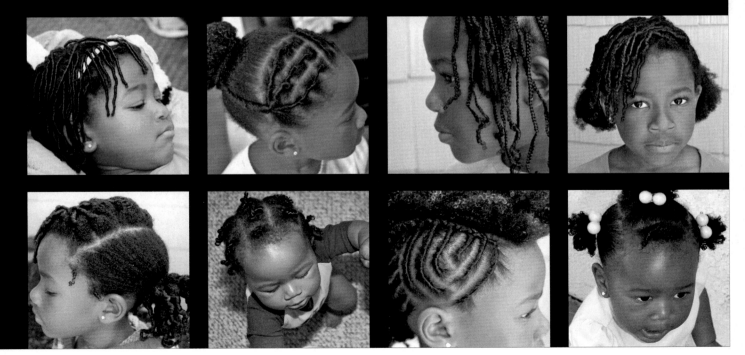

TWO-STRAND TWISTS

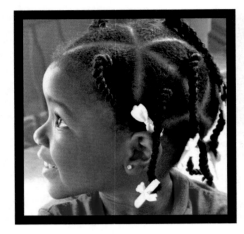 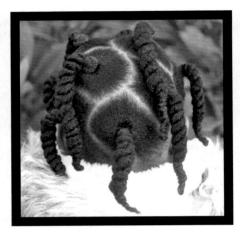 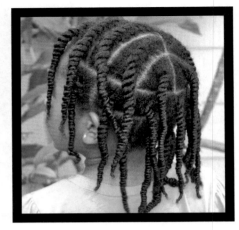

Whereas coils are created from a single section of hair, two-strand twists are formed from two sections of hair that are twisted over one another. When working your way into new styling techniques, twists are an excellent step up from coils. They do, however, require a certain amount of length, texture, and curl pattern in order to hold their shape. Two-strand twists can also be used to form a twist-out, which is a hairstyle created by setting the hair into twists until it dries and then unraveling, to leave behind a curl-like pattern. The size of the twists will dictate the pattern of the twist-out.

Twists are a great way to keep the hair moisturized and detangled. They also form a nice base to more advanced styles like pinned rosettes and Bantu knots. Twists can be used for both boys and girls, although rope twists are used almost exclusively for girls.

REGULAR TWISTS VERSUS ROPE TWISTS

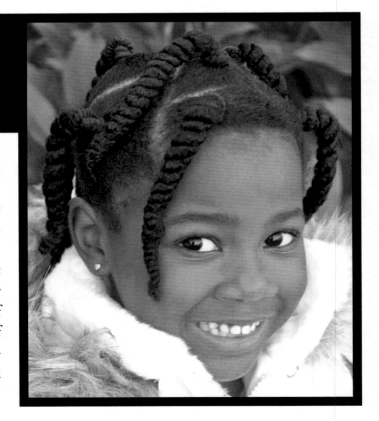

Twists can be formed in the traditional way by just wrapping one section over the other to make "regular" twists. Or, they can be done as "rope" twists, where the individual strands are twisted in one direction *prior* to being twisted over one another in the *opposite direction*. Regular twists are faster to style than rope twists, but do not have as much definition and tend to get fuzzier more quickly. In addition, given the same amount of hair, the diameter of rope twists is smaller than that of regular twists. **NOTE:** Although the following tutorials illustrate twisting right-over-left, you can twist in whichever direction is most comfortable for you.

Regular Twists Two-Strand

- Leave-in Conditioner
- Moisturizer (for thick/coarse hair)
- Sealing Oil or Butter
- Styling Gel or Cream (optional)

Form regular twists by wrapping one section of the hair over another (left-over-right or right-over-left). In this tutorial, notice that the individual strands of yarn are visible in each section as they're being twisted; this is why regular twists do not appear as shiny as rope twists, and why the hair is likely to become fuzzy more quickly.

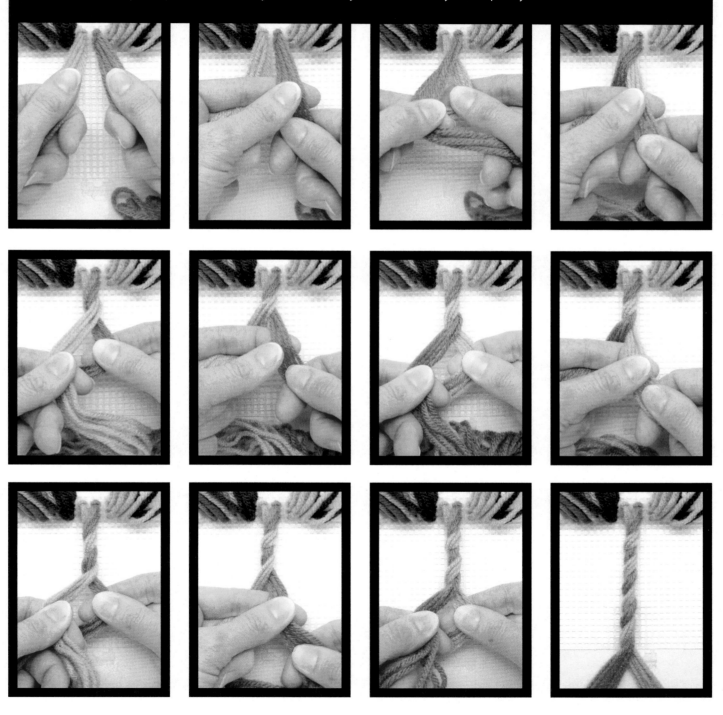

Rope Twists Two-Strand

- Leave-in Conditioner
- Moisturizer (for thick/coarse hair)
- Sealing Oil or Butter
- Styling Gel or Cream (optional)

Rope twists are formed from two sections; however the right-hand section is coiled *clockwise* before passing it over the left-hand section *counter-clockwise*. As the left-hand section is passes beneath the coiled right-hand section, it becomes the *new* right-hand section that you coil, repeating the previous steps.

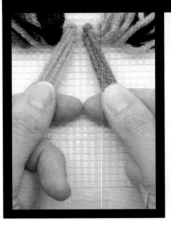
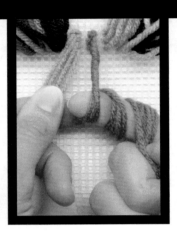
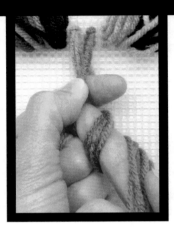
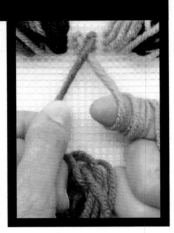

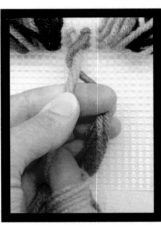
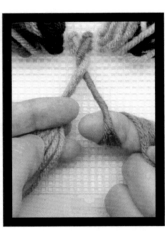
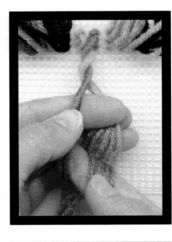
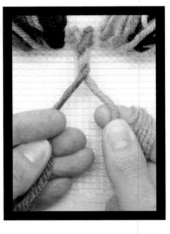

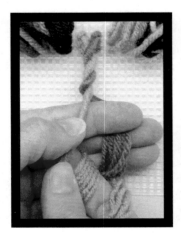
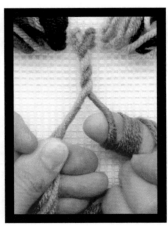
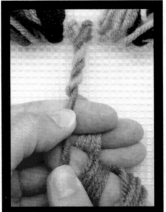
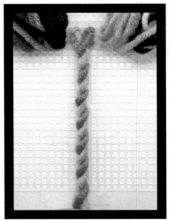

| CHOCOLATE HAIR VANILLA CARE
A Parent's Guide to
Beginning Natural Hair Styling

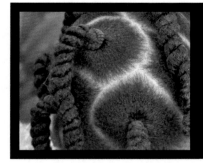

REGULAR or ROPE Twists?

Because rope twists are pre-twisted when formed, they are both smaller in diameter and shinier than regular twists.

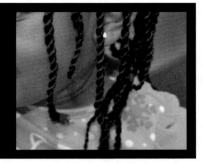

When **REGULAR** Twists May Be Preferable

- When you want twists that are quicker to style.
- When your child has thinner or finer hair, and you want the twists to fill in the hairstyle.
- When you want to do a twist-out on thin or fine hair.
- When a style that is not perfectly fuzz-free is okay and you're not planning on leaving it in for too long.
- When you want twists with a larger diameter.

When **ROPE** Twists May Be Preferable

- When you have the time to invest in more defined twists.
- When your child's hair is really thick or coarse, and you want your twists to hang more freely.
- When you want a well-defined twist-out, and your child has enough hair to fill in with rope twists.
- When you want a sleeker, more fuzz-free look and you plan on leaving the style in for a while.
- When you want a thinner diameter to the twists.

TWIST STYLES

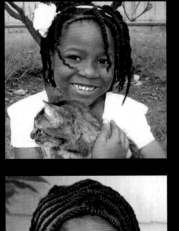
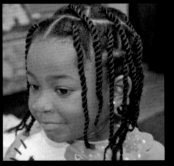
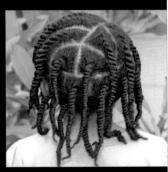
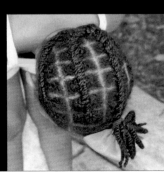
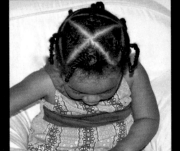
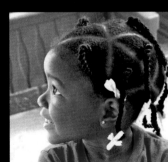

THREE-STRAND BRAIDS OR "SINGLES"

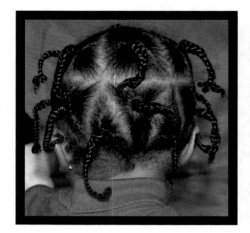 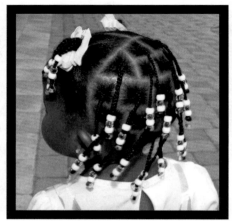 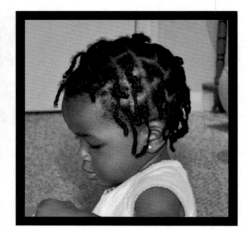

Braids are the most universally known styling technique, even for those who are otherwise unfamiliar with natural hair. They are formed by weaving three sections of hair in a pattern so that the hair stays both detangled and moisturized.

Box braids, also known as "singles," are hanging braids formed from several sections usually parted in a pattern, or "boxes." The smaller the boxes, the smaller the braids will be; and the smaller the braids, the longer they take to remove when restyling.

OVERHAND BRAIDING VERSUS UNDERHAND BRAIDING

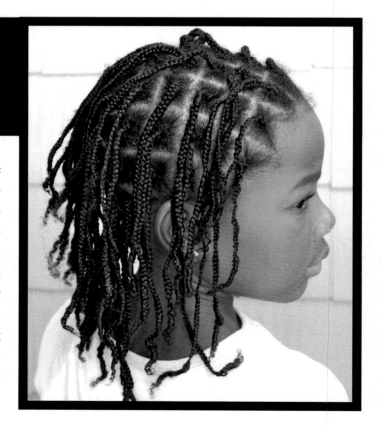

The braiding tutorials on the next two pages illustrate how to form a three-strand braid using both the overhand and the underhand methods. If you know how to French braid, then you are already familiar with overhand braiding. Understanding the difference between forming underhand and overhand braids is essential when learning how to cornrow. Cornrows are similar to French braids with one major difference: They are an *underhand* braid. If you can master underhand braiding with your box braids, learning to cornrow will be much easier. If your child is still a baby or toddler, now is the perfect time to practice.

- Leave-in Conditioner
- Moisturizer (for thick/coarse hair)
- Sealing Oil or Butter
- Styling Gel or Cream (optional)

Begin by dividing the hair into three sections. Select either the left or right section and pass it OVER the center section, then repeat the step on the opposite side. In overhand braiding, the outside sections are alternately crossing OVER the center section, becoming the new center section each time.

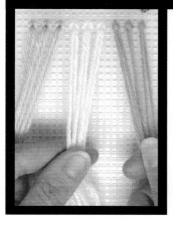
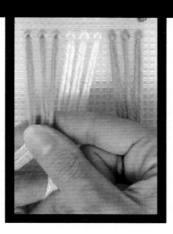
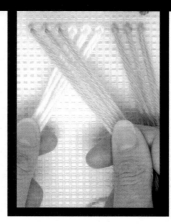
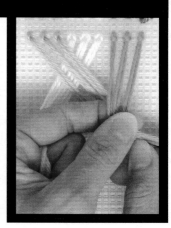

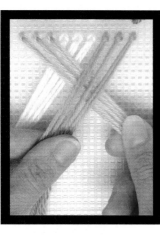
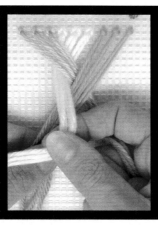
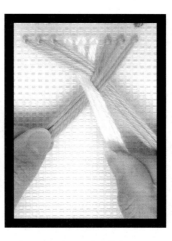
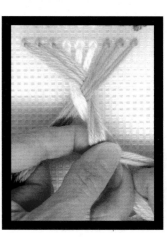

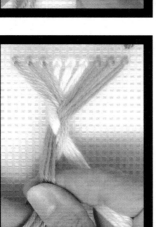
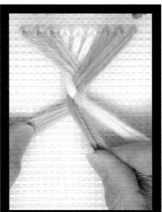
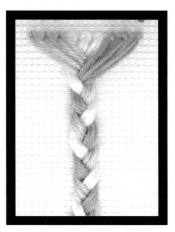

Braiding Underhand

PRODUCTS

- Leave-in Conditioner
- Moisturizer (for thick/coarse hair)
- Sealing Oil or Butter
- Styling Gel or Cream (optional)

Begin by dividing the hair into three sections. Select either the left or right section and pass it UNDER the center section, then repeat the step on the opposite side. In underhand braiding, the outside sections are alternately crossing UNDER the center section, becoming the new center section each time.

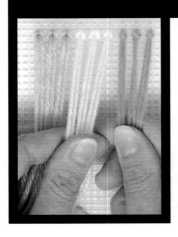 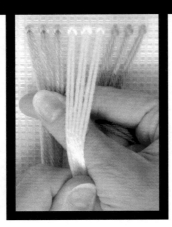 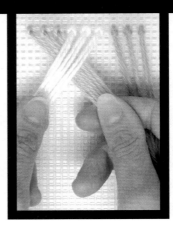 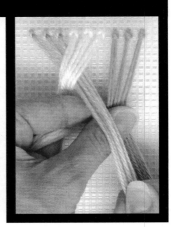

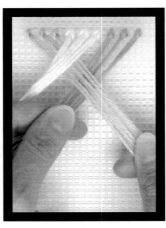 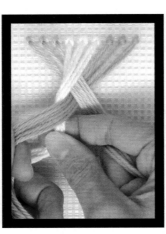 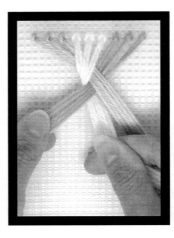 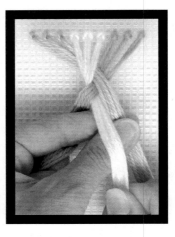

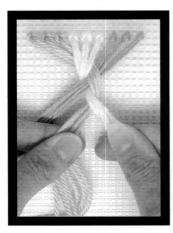 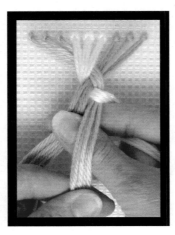 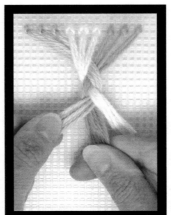 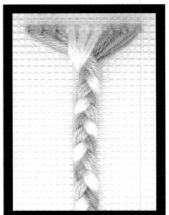

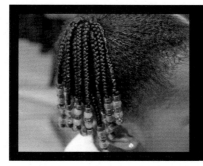

BRAIDS or TWISTS?

A box braid has a top and a bottom, whereas twists are round with no distinct "side." Thus, braids will lay flush on top of one another.

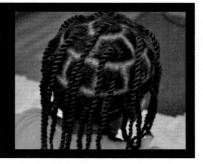

When **BRAIDS** May Be Preferable

- When working with hair that is finer in texture.
- When you want a flatter look to the hair in your boxes.
- When you braid more quickly than you twist and time is important.
- When braids hold your child's hair better than twists.
- When you want to style a braid-out.
- When the time it takes to remove the braids is not an issue.

When **TWISTS** May Be Preferable

- When the curl pattern and texture of the hair hold better in twists than in braids.
- When you want the hair in the boxes to be chunkier.
- When you twist faster than you braid, and time is important.
- When you want to style a twist-out.
- When you don't want to invest the time it takes to remove braids.

BRAID STYLES

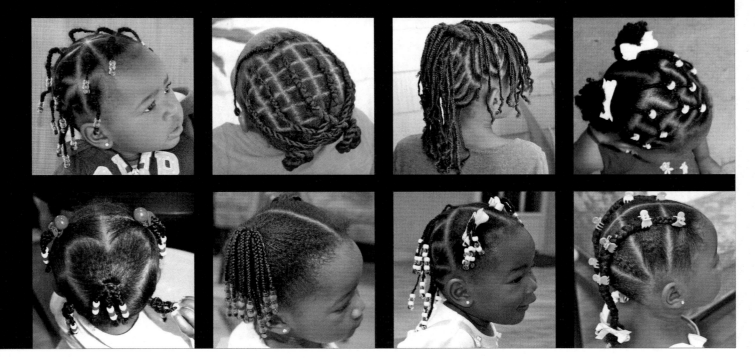

Finishing Box Braids & Twists

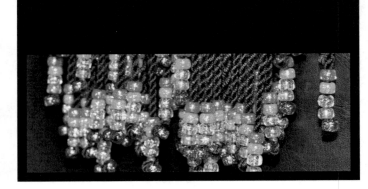

So you've parted some boxes and you've styled some nice braids or twists. Do you need to put anything on the bottom of these box styles to keep them from coming unraveled? The answer depends on any number of factors, including your skill level, the tightness of the curl pattern, the texture of the hair, your child's activity level, how you protect the hair while styled, and the maturity level of your little one (*e.g.*, whether or not your child will pull out accessories). Generally speaking, the coarser the hair texture and the tighter the curl pattern, the less likely you will need to put something on the ends. A good holding product, smaller boxes, and tighter braids or twists can all assist with keeping them from coming undone. Below are additional options.

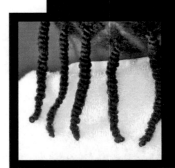

NOTHING

Ideally, to minimize breakage, you do not want to use any accessories on the ends, especially if the hair will hold the braid or twist on its own.

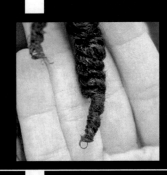

COILS

Coils are a great way to finish the ends of braids or twists, especially if the ends are too uneven to finish toward the bottom.

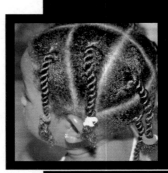

BANDS

Bands of any variety can be used to finish box braids and twists. Keep in mind product warnings regarding choking hazards.

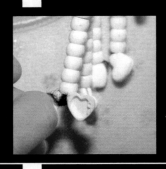

SNAPS

If you want to avoid elastics, snaps are specifically designed to finish off the ends of box braids and twists, especially when using beads.

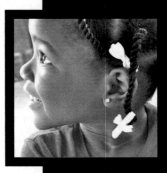

BARRETTES

Twisting the ends of your boxes around a plastic barrette is another option, especially for younger kids. Do note that barrettes do not hold as well in finer hair.

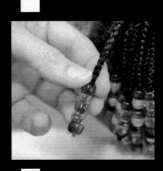

BEADS

Beads are another way to hide the uneven ends of box braids and twists, but require something to secure them to the hair (*e.g.*, elastics, snaps, or barrettes).

To Band or Not to Band

In a perfect world, nicely parted box twists or singles would stay secured at the base and ends without the need for bands. However, this is less likely with thinner or finer hair. True protective styling does not use anything that can cause tension breakage, but sometimes it's necessary to find the right balance between promoting hair growth and using helpers. Only you will know whether or not your child's hair can tolerate bands; I used them when my daughter was younger, but moved away from them as her curl pattern tightened and they became unnecessary.

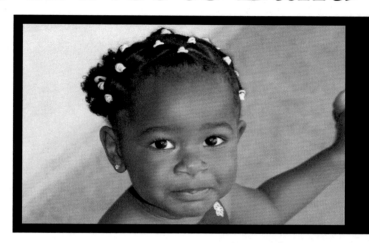

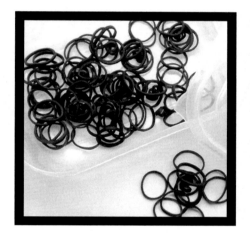

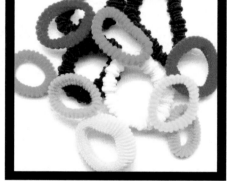

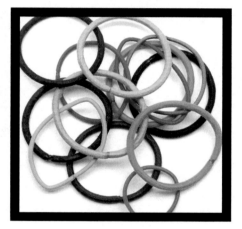

RUBBER BANDS

Rubber bands, also referred to as elastics, are the items to which I'm generally referring when talking about securing the base or ends of small box braids, or when securing beads. Although often a favorite for securing fine hairs on babies and toddlers, they can break easily (especially when used in conjunction with hair products) and become a choking hazard. Please follow the age recommendations on packaging and use your discretion. Small children often pull on their box braids and twists and can easily remove them.

TERRYCLOTH O's

Terrycloth O's are a favorite for banding the base of larger sections of hair to form chunky twists and braids. They do not provide the same amount of tension as rubber bands or pony O's, but they don't cause as much breakage as a result. Generally, the elastic does not last more than a few uses. Therefore, if you invest in them, know that they will stretch out quickly and need to be replaced often. That being said, they are relatively inexpensive and are my go-to band when I'm stretching the hair before styling.

PONY O's

Pony O's are made specifically to hold ponytails and puffs, usually in larger quantities of hair than in boxes. You can find them in smaller sizes, but the elasticity and flexibility can usually be better served by rubber bands or terrycloth O's. Pony O's provide a great deal of tension when wrapped several times, which is great for holding larger puffs, but can also pull too tightly on finer hair or fragile edges, causing breakage. If you use them for sock buns and puffs, try to mix up the styles so that the hair is not under constant tension, and the scalp gets a break.

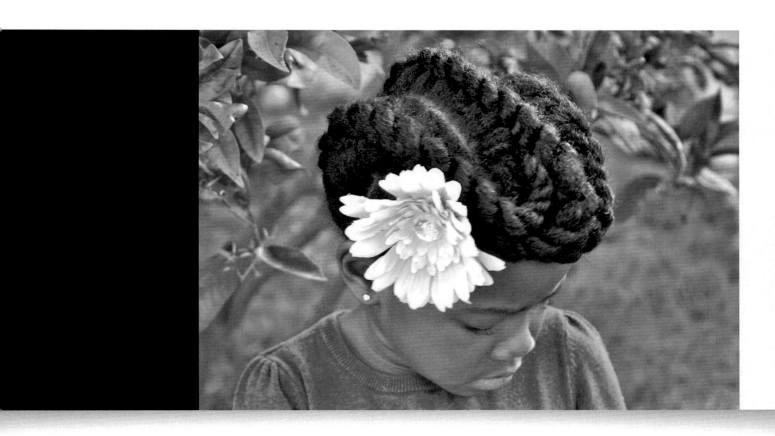

PART IV
FLAT BRAIDS & FLAT TWISTS

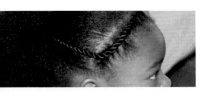
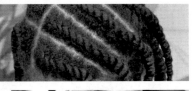
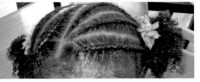

OVERVIEW OF FLAT BRAIDS & FLAT TWISTS

Flat braids and twists don't have to be done in tiny little sections, nor do they need to cover the entire head. The joy of learning how to do different hairstyles is choosing to mix and match techniques that meet your family's needs as well as your skill level. I've come up with some of my most creative designs after "throwing in the towel" on a new technique and finishing the hairstyle with a method in which I was both quicker and more confident.

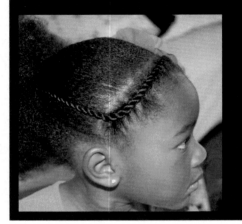 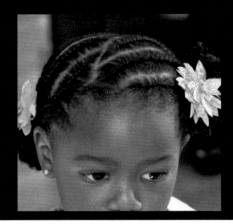 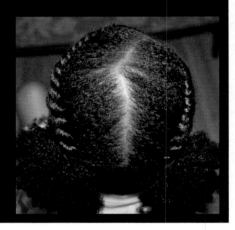

Cornrows (the type of flat braid used most in this book) and flat twists are both excellent protective hairstyles because they do a great job of addressing common issues related to moisture loss and breakage. Since these styles keep the hair close to the scalp, they help reduce friction and exposure to the elements while also minimizing the need to draw them up into a ponytail or finish the ends with anything that could cause breakage.

Learning to cornrow and flat twist is a process that will take time; just know that you do not have to form tiny rows of numerous cornrows or flat twists your first time around. In fact, the best way to approach learning these techniques is to choose a style that requires only one or two rows. If you feel the need to redo your cornrow or flat twist, removing one is much easier than removing several. In addition, using fewer rows is an easy way to practice parting without becoming overwhelmed with the need to complete a full head of them. As you get quicker and more confident, you can try increasing the number or decreasing the width of your rows, taking into account how long your child is willing to sit for you.

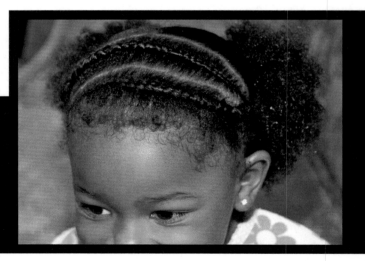

START SIMPLE

Completing one or two cornrows or flat twists is a great way to get the practice you need as both you and your child learn to work together for styling.

FLAT TWISTS

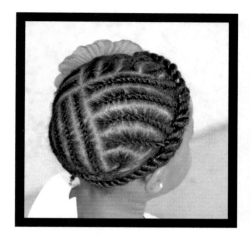 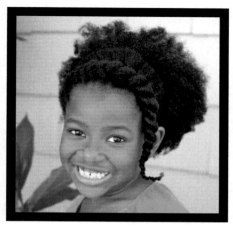 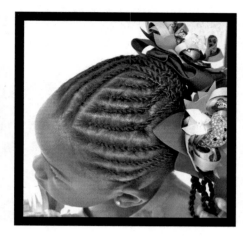

Flat twists go by a variety of names, depending on whom you ask. For the sake of simplicity, I will refer to flat twists as a type of row formed from twisting two alternating sections of hair over one another, adding hair to each section as you go. I will cover both regular flat twists and flat rope twists, much like I did for boxed twists. If you've already mastered boxed twists, these flat sister-versions will likely come more easily to you.

If you are entirely new to hair braiding, you may want to start with twists over braids, and flat twists over cornrows. The simplicity of working with only two sections makes them an ideal option for anyone unaccustomed to holding sections of hair in their hands. Once you've learned how to grasp two sections, twisting and adding more hair as you go, braiding with three sections would be the next logical step.

CHOOSING A TWISTING DIRECTION TO ACHIEVE A PREFERRED LOOK

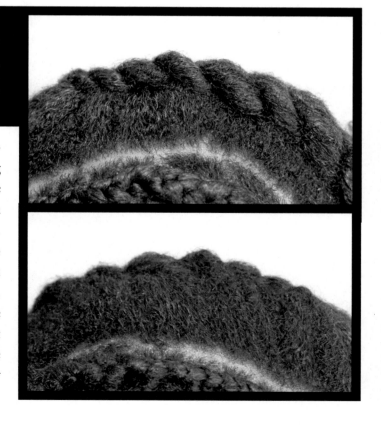

Although flat twists may be easier to learn than cornrows, the fact that they have a "side" may seem confusing to people new to styling. When braiding a cornrow, the row is flat and appears the same when looking at it from both sides of the row. This is not the case with flat twists. The two photos to the right illustrate this point: The top photo is a flat twist as seen from one side; the bottom photo is the *same flat twist* as seen from the *opposite* side. Flat twists will usually have more definition on the side to which you're twisting. So if you are forming a twist right-over-left, the left-hand side of the twist will be more defined than the right-hand side. This discrepancy is usually more noticeable with flat rope twists.

Regular Flat Twists

PRODUCTS

- Leave-in Conditioner
- Moisturizer (for thick/coarse hair)
- Sealing Oil or Butter
- Styling Gel or Cream (optional)

Regular flat twists are formed by taking one section of hair and passing it over another, adding hair each time as you move down the row. The tighter you form your twist, the more the hair sections will blend into one another. Looser flat twists will show the individual sections wrapping over one another more clearly.

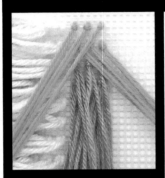

Start your twist with two sections.

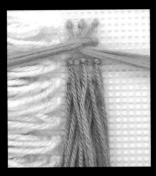

Swap the two sections, right over left.

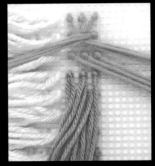

Add hair to the new right section.

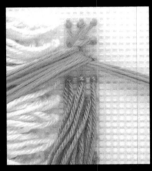

Swap the two sections, right over left.

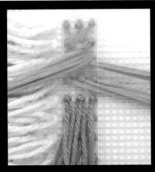

Add hair to the new right section.

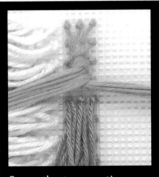

Swap the two sections, right over left.

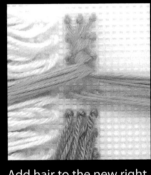

Add hair to the new right section.

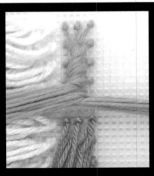

Swap the two sections, right over left.

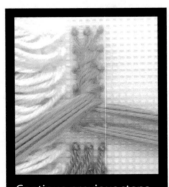

Continue previous steps until row is completed.

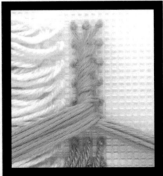

The row is getting longer and thicker.

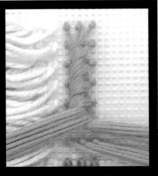

Notice you can still see the individual strands.

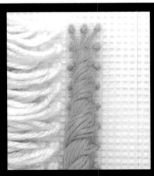

The finished flat twist will be raised off the scalp.

PRODUCTS

- Leave-in Conditioner
- Moisturizer (for thick/coarse hair)
- Sealing Oil or Butter
- Styling Gel or Cream

What makes these different from regular flat twists is that the hair is coiled together in one direction on the side to which it is being added *before* it is passed over to the *opposite* side. The photos below illustrate a twist that is going toward the left-hand side, which means the left-hand side will be more defined than the right.

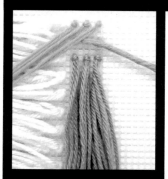

Pre-twist your right section toward the right.

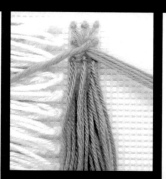

Swap the two sections, right over left.

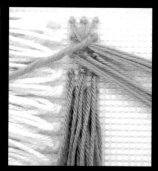

Add hair to the new right section.

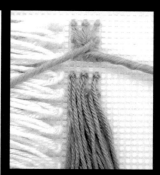

Pre-twist the new right section toward the right.

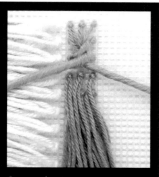

Swap the two sections, right over left.

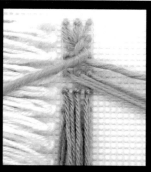

Add hair to the new right section.

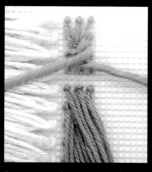

Pre-twist the new right section toward the right.

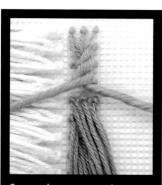

Swap the two sections, right over left.

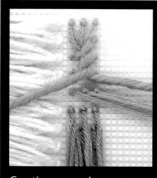

Continue previous steps until row is completed.

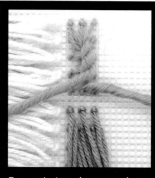

Pre-twisting the strands adds definition to the row.

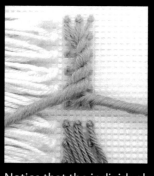

Notice that the individual strands are blended.

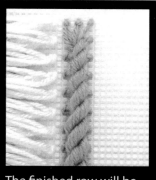

The finished row will be defined and raised.

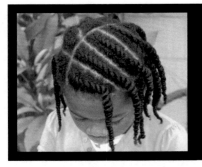

REGULAR Flat Twists or Flat ROPE Twists?

Flat twists are quick and easy but do not last nearly as long as flat rope twists.

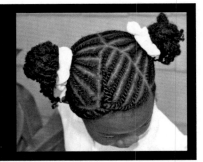

When REGULAR Flat Twists May Be Preferable

- When the definition of the individual stitches is not that important to the style.
- When you have less time to style.
- When you're not planning on leaving the style in for a long time or you're tolerant of a few fuzzies.
- When your child's scalp is easily stressed with any level of tension.
- When you want thicker twists that sit further off the scalp.

When Flat ROPE Twists May Be Preferable

- When you want to see the definition of the rope pattern along the individual rows.
- When you have the time to do the pre-twisting step.
- When you want the hairstyle to look sleeker and more defined for a longer period of time.
- When you know that your child's scalp can handle a bit of tension without causing stress.
- When you want thinner twists that sit closer to the scalp.

FLAT TWIST STYLES

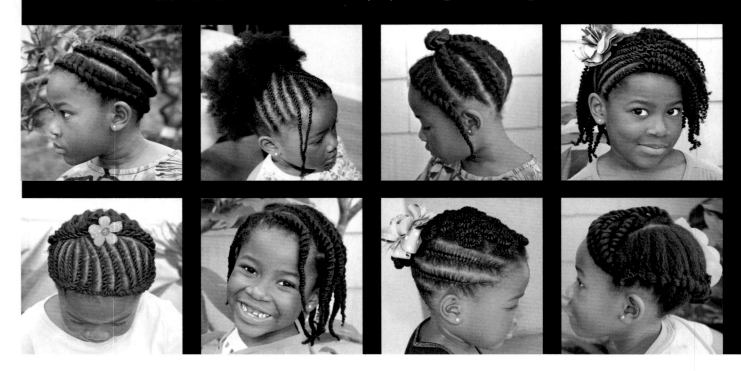

CORNROWS

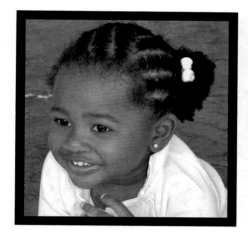
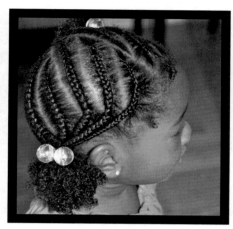
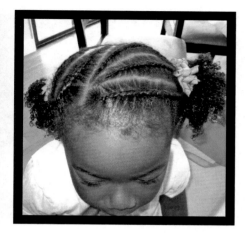

Many believe cornrows are just smaller versions of French braids. This, however, is untrue. As I mentioned in Part III, a cornrow is an *underhand* braid, and a French braid is an *overhand* braid. Cornrows create braids that sit on top of the row; French braids are usually more loose and inverted, so that the braid is hidden beneath the stitches. The *size* of the braid itself has no bearing on what *type* of braid it is.

Flat braid types are defined by two characteristics: Overhand versus underhand, and to which section the hair is added while braiding. Cornrows are not the only underhand braid: Dutch braids are also an underhand braid; in fact, many use the two interchangeably on natural hair. For a true cornrow, hair is added to the *middle* section as you are braiding, but for Dutch braids, hair is added to the *outer* sections.

USING BOX BRAIDS TO PRACTICE CORNROWS

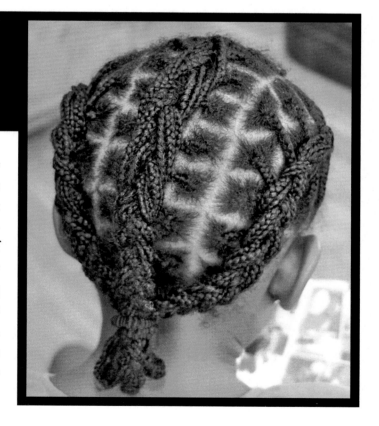

Creating a practice board for braiding is a great way to learn how to do cornrows. However, if you lack the time or inclination to do so, you can always use box braids to hone your technique. Working with reasonably small boxes, the braids provide pre-sized chunks of hair with which to work. In addition, they are also easy to remove if you make a mistake. Further, cornrowing your boxed braids is yet another styling option if you're looking to add variety. In the photo to the right, I did three cornrows in my daughter's hair, starting in the front and moving toward the back, finishing with a terrycloth O to keep the ends tucked under for swimming.

Cornrows

- Leave-in Conditioner
- Moisturizer (for thick/coarse hair)
- Sealing Oil or Butter
- Styling Gel or Cream

Cornrows are formed by doing an underhand three-strand braid, adding hair to the middle section as you move down the length of the row. Although tension is helpful to preserve the style, too much tension can stress the scalp and possibly lead to breakage. If you see any puckering of the scalp between the stitches, the rows are too tight.

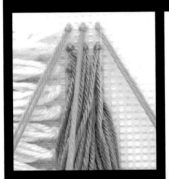

Part one row into three sections.

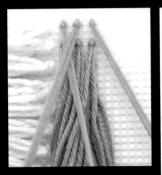

Swap left section under center.

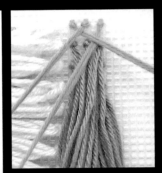

Swap right section under center.

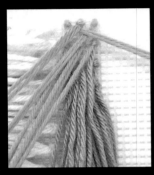

Add hair to center section.

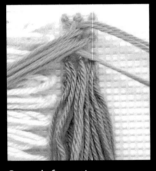

Swap left section under center.

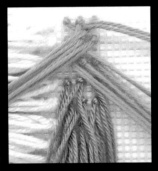

Add hair to center section.

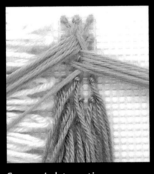

Swap right section under center.

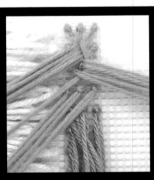

Add hair to center section.

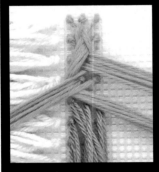

Swap left section under center.

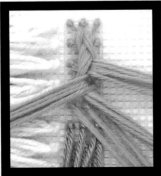

Continue previous steps until row is completed.

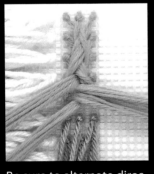

Be sure to alternate direction of center section.

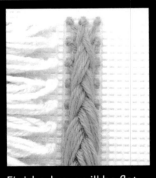

Finished row will be flat and close to scalp.

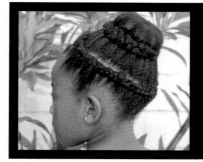

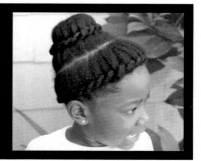

CORNROWS or FLAT TWISTS?

Cornrows lay flat along the scalp with no discernible side; flat twists are raised and have a "direction."

When **CORNROWS** May Be Preferable

- When your child's hair holds better in braids, and hairstyle longevity is important to you.
- When the style will benefit from having flatter rows.
- When you want the hairstyle to look the same from all directions.
- When you cornrow faster than flat twist, and efficiency is important to you.
- When you know you'll have the time to remove the style.

When **FLAT TWISTS** May Be Preferable

- When your child's hair holds better in twists, and hairstyle longevity is important to you.
- When the style looks better with rows that "pop."
- When the design you're doing dictates that the hair be more defined from one angle over another.
- When you flat twist faster than cornrow, and efficiency is important to you.
- When you want a style that takes less time to
- remove.

CORNROW STYLES

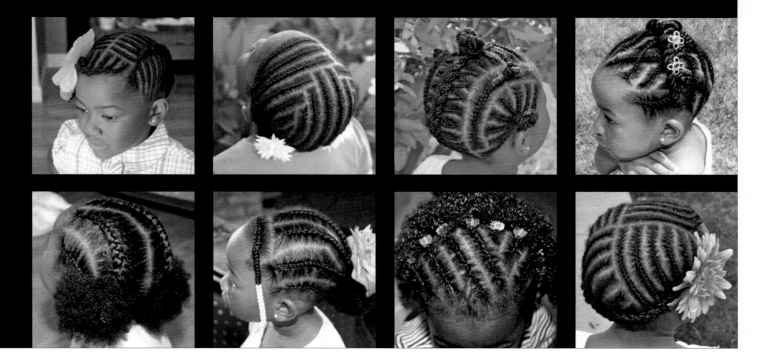

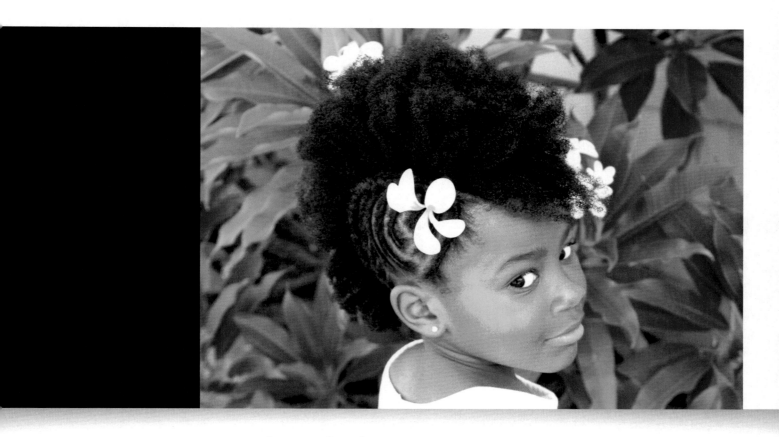

PART V
HAIRSTYLING

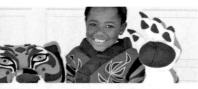
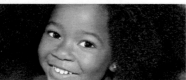
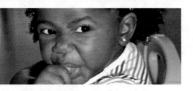
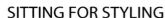

OUTLINING STYLING NEEDS

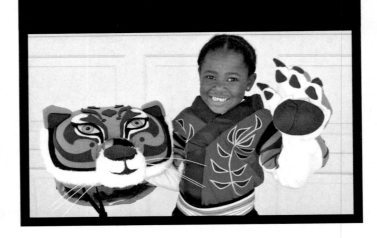

Just because you *can* do amazing things with natural hair, does it mean that you *should?* The answer boils down to your styling needs. Determining what you and your child want when it comes to hair care will help you better decide how much, or how little, styling is necessary. If you plan on keeping your child's hair cut short (especially for boys), there's really no need to focus on styling that promotes length retention. In addition, if you're planning on locking your child's hair as soon as it's long enough to do so, then teaching her to sit for long hours of styling would likely not be an efficient use of family time. A variety of factors go into assessing styling needs and can range from issues related to the entire family (*e.g.,* time and skill level of the person styling) to individual needs (*e.g.,* a child's desire to have long hair like her siblings). It's a delicate balancing act. Only you will be able to determine the needs specific to your own family. What follows are a few items to consider.

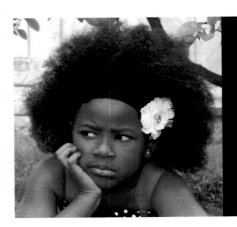

TIME MANAGEMENT

If you feel like you're spending too much time detangling, or that the daily upkeep of free hair is becoming overwhelming for you or your child, a protective hairstyle can help. Learning to style the hair in ways that keep it detangled between wash days can free up time on busy school mornings, as well as minimize the time it takes to wash and detangle the hair. This is especially something to consider if you have several children and a very busy daily schedule.

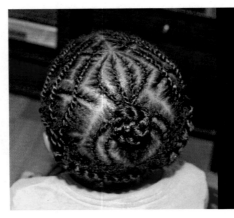

HAIRSTYLE LONGEVITY EXPECTATIONS

Determine how long you would like the hairstyle to last. Do you have a vacation coming up? Will you be traveling and unavailable to do hair? Do you have plans the next few weekends that would prohibit your ability to do hair? If so, the time invested in setting a more complicated protective hairstyle can give you and your child the freedom to enjoy upcoming activities without having to worry about working styling into an already busy schedule.

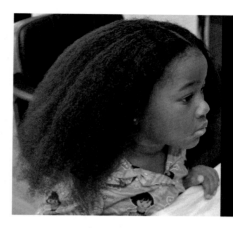

OVERALL HAIR GOALS

Generally speaking, it's very unlikely that your child will be able to wear her hair without any styling if the overall goal is to grow hair as long as possible. Styling protects against moisture loss and breakage; the tighter the curl pattern, the more difficult it can be to grow hair from the root faster than it breaks off on the ends. If long hair is the goal, protective styling that keeps the ends from breaking off will help with length retention.

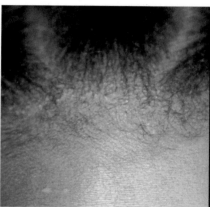

HAIR & SCALP ISSUES

Is your child's scalp always dry? Does it stress out easily with just minor tension? These are things to consider when styling. There is no need to do cornrows on a scalp that doesn't tolerate them. There are plenty of other options that will help achieve the same goals. However, if your child's scalp is always dry, nice rows can help you identify trouble spots and address them more easily. Furthermore, if your child's hair is prone to dryness and breakage, good styling can help your moisturizing products work better.

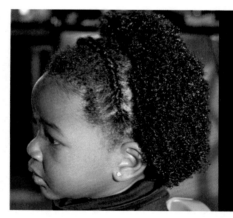

PROTECTING EDGES

If your child's hair is still filling in along the hairline, or if your older child has been experiencing breakage, selecting styles that do not pull on the hairline would be ideal. This includes avoiding headbands that rub the affected areas. If protecting edges is an issue and long hair is a goal, try to select hairstyles that do not pull on them. Avoid puffs and buns (or pulling boxed styles up into ponytails) and do your flat twists and cornrows *toward* the hairline instead of away from it.

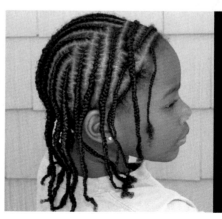

BOY HAIRSTYLES

If you have a boy, all of the above issues still apply. It all comes down to what your goals are and then deciding on the right path toward achieving them. Some hairstyles look better on girls than boys; where exactly that line is drawn often varies depending on where you live. Some locales are more accepting than others when it comes to boys with certain hairstyles. Don't know what's acceptable in your area? Take a look around. And ask questions. Get your cues from your community.

GETTING YOUR CHILD INVOLVED

Although it may seem intuitive, involving your child in the process of her own hair care goes a long way in how compliant she will be during styling. Not only are you, the "stylist," learning about natural hair, you are the one who will ultimately become your child's teacher, passing along your newfound information.

For babies and toddlers, obviously you will be making the majority of the choices. However, the earlier you give children options, the more empowered they will feel. Hairstyling becomes less of a chore when it's an activity agreed upon by *all* parties involved.

Children's opinions seem to be directly proportional to their age, so the older they get, the stronger they may feel about certain hairstyling choices. Selecting how their hair is styled is just another form of expressing their in-dividual personalities. On occasion, you will likely disagree with their choices, so fostering good communication early can help mitigate those disagreements. Should conflict arise, the better you *both* understand the process of styling, the easier it will be to express your views and reach a solution.

In short, knowledge is not only power for you, the caregiver doing the hair, but also empowerment for your child. Remember that it is your child who will ultimately be wearing the hairstyle. Again, hairstyling is a delicate balancing act between the wants and needs of all involved. Try to keep that in mind when selecting a hairstyle, especially if the style requires that your child curb her normal play or activities, or if she feels it doesn't reflect her personality.

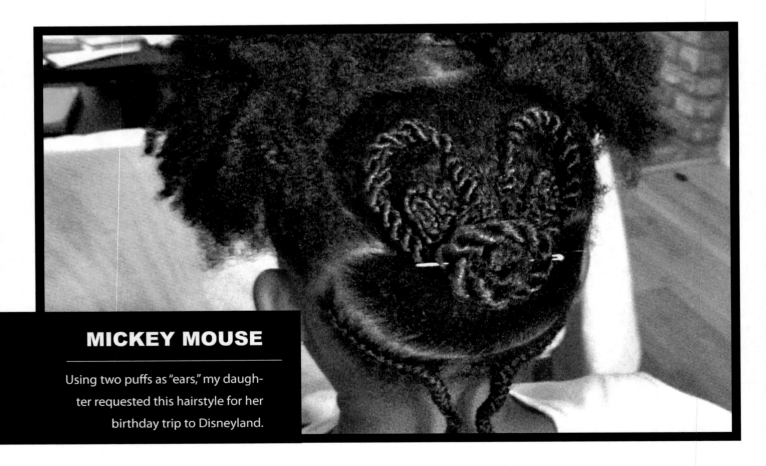

MICKEY MOUSE

Using two puffs as "ears," my daughter requested this hairstyle for her birthday trip to Disneyland.

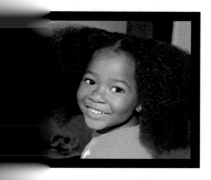

AGREE ON HAIR GOALS

Agreeing on hair goals is the number one thing that needs to happen before styling. If you want your child to have long, healthy hair, but she couldn't care less about length, you will likely have problems when it comes to styling; a child who doesn't care isn't going to see the value in sitting for styling. When your child is younger, you will have more of a say. However, if your child begins to dread styling, perhaps it's time to reassess the overall hair goals.

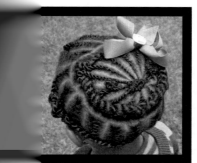

GIVE YOUR CHILD OPTIONS

I give my daughter a great deal of freedom when it comes to requesting hairstyles because I'm willing to try just about anything. However, I have limits on when we do this (usually only during the summer). If your child requests a hairstyle that challenges your abilities, she will likely be more patient while you're trying because she feels heard. Even if it doesn't turn out exactly how your child (or you) wanted, at the very least you've built trust by fostering an open a path of communication.

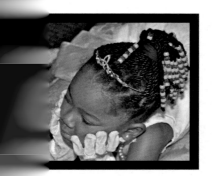

ASK FOR INPUT ON ACCESSORIES

Did you just buy a new package of beads? Did your daughter get a set of bows for her birthday? Does she want to go to that princess party at her friend's house? Sometimes your child will let you do just about any style *you* want, just as long as she can wear that accessory *she* wants in her hair. That being said, be sure to keep in mind upcoming events and whether or not she's going to want to change out accessories over the duration of the style.

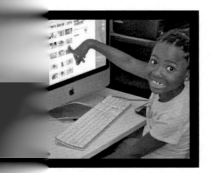

OUTLINE PROCESS BEFOREHAND

Letting your child know what to expect ahead of time will help avoid conflict during the process. If you're doing a head full of boxes or rows, tell her how many you would like to complete before the first break. Then keep her informed as you're working. Make a math game out of it. Just let her know what's coming and when to expect breaks. Try making a hairstyle selection together, discussing how long you think it will take, and how you plan on breaking the process up to get it done.

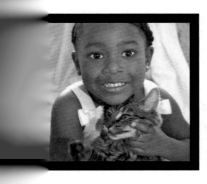

BE FLEXIBLE

So you've outlined the hair process and then something happens and you have to alter the plan. Roll with it. It's going to happen. It may be something small (like getting distracted by a family pet), or it may become clear that your child is getting sick and needs to stop. Perhaps you need to leave the house for a family emergency and you're in the middle of styling. Grab a scarf, wrap it up, and go. Life happens, and hair is just a teeny, tiny part of it. If you remember to keep styling in perspective, so will your child.

SETTING REALISTIC EXPECTATIONS

Preparation goes a long way for both you and your child. We started styling with a pretty rigid hair care routine that has since become more flexible as my daughter has grown and my skills have increased. What works for one age may not work as your child gets older. Perhaps your family has grown—maybe you've become a single parent or have returned to the workforce. Things happen in life and, just like any other part of child-rearing, hairstyling will just have to roll with it.

Though you can't control the future, you can set realistic expectations for the present. Those expectations need to be clear to both you and your child in order for them to be most effective. Each styling session will be different. You may be doing a hairstyle you've done before, but a variety of external factors may have changed. Set your expectations for that session specifically, rather than a general expectation of how all sessions should go.

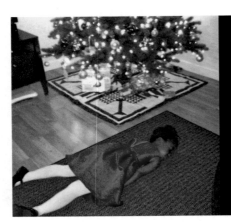

TIME COMMITMENT

If you don't want to feel rushed during styling, try to avoid time crunches. Know how much time you have to commit and plan accordingly. I've found that the holidays are toughest for us because my daughter's birthday is also in December; a long-lasting protective hairstyle done once or twice between Halloween and the New Year works best for us at that time of year. Expecting to squeeze a complicated hairstyle into a busy schedule will likely be unrealistic, so plan ahead.

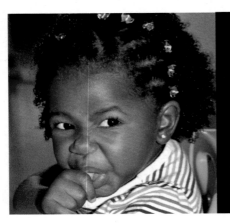

MOOD

If you didn't sleep well the night before, or if you are sick or otherwise not feeling well, it's unrealistic to expect that you're going to be your best during styling. This is true for your child as well. There are some circumstances in life that you cannot control; but when you *can* control them, it helps to do so to avoid conflict. If my child is sick, she will usually be fine with sitting for a longer style because she doesn't feel like playing; if she's full of energy, I'm likely going to have a squirmy kid on my hands.

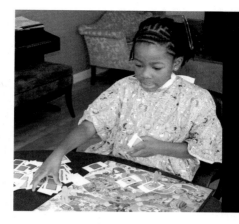

ENTERTAINMENT

Plan on more distractions and entertainment for your child than you think you will ever realistically need. It's better to have too many options than to run out of things to do in the middle of a session. I like to reserve some special activities that are exclusively used during hairstyling (like watching television or a movie). Styling becomes a treat when your child gets to do something that she enjoys, especially if she can *only* do it when getting her hair done.

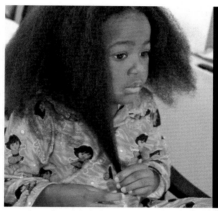

PERSONALITIES

Some kids are just more fidgety than others, and that's totally okay. If you're styling more than one head of hair, just keep in mind that what works for one child may not work for another. Cater to each child's personality, both to avoid conflict with that child and to foster trust and communication. As your children get older, they will hopefully appreciate your acknowledgment of their different personalities. This is especially important if you have children with any special needs.

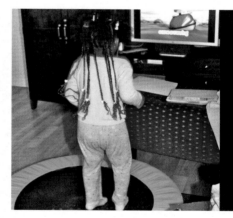

BREAKS

Yes, you may want to work through styling with no breaks, but your child is young and will need to move often. We call it "getting the wiggles out," taking breaks often during styling. Schedule them. Plan on them. Expect to need them when you're right in the middle of a very complicated part. If you expect interruptions at any moment, you will be less frustrated when the need for one arises. Less frustration equals more enjoyable, quality hair time.

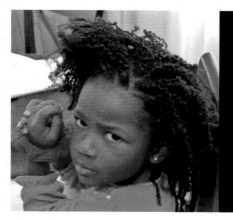

ATTITUDE

Sometimes parents get so caught up in doing hair that they forget to take it one step further, from a neutral experience to a positive experience. A touch, a word, a laugh, a smile, all of those will imprint on your little one and help her form a lasting, healthy relationship with her own hair. Even when I feel like I don't know what I'm doing, or I'm afraid I'm going to mess something up, it's funny how acting positive about my daughter's hair for *her* sake rubs out my *own* fears of inadequacy.

SITTING FOR STYLING

Although some children may be able to focus for longer periods of time, there is nothing magical about having a child sit to have her hair done. But like anything we teach our children, it's a process that happens over a period of time. Only you know your child's personality; nobody can tell you how long you should expect your child to sit. However, if you've been honing your styling skills and have been including your child in the process, taking into account all of the factors mentioned in the previous sections, your child will likely learn to sit for increasingly longer periods of time.

Start touching your child's hair in a "styling" way as early as you can, in short periods to help gauge personality and trust; it will help you assess how much your child can handle. If your child is a baby and you're just learning how to care for natural hair, you will both grow accustomed to styling at the same time. You will get faster and more skilled, and your child will get better at sitting for you.

For an older child who has just joined the family, including her in as much of the process as possible is of paramount importance. Look at pictures with her and talk about what your child wants. She may never have had her hair done before, so it will be a learning process for you both. If she has had her hair styled before, ask about what those experiences were like and what her expectations are. Giving her a voice in the process will do wonders in fostering a healthy self-image.

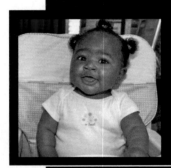

Booster Seat

Use a high chair or booster seat if your child is really young so that she learns to stay in one place during styling.

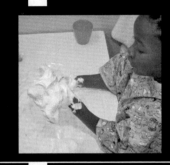

Sink Play

Styling your child while sitting at the sink opens up a world of water play, including playing with shaving cream.

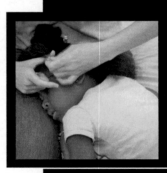

While Sleeping

Although doing hair while sleeping does not teach your child to sit for styling, it's still a reasonable option, especially for babies and toddlers.

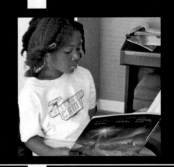

While Reading

For the avid reader, there's nothing like a getting lost in a good book to make styling time fly by.

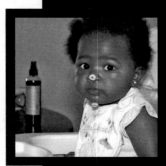

While Eating

Taking snack time to spritz hair and try out some coils is a great way to keep babies and toddlers distracted.

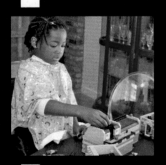

Playing Legos

Legos are fun because they can work on a table or in your child's lap and have endless possibilities for creative play.

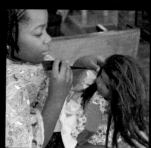

Styling Dolls

While I'm styling my daughter's hair, she likes to style her "daughter's" hair, too.

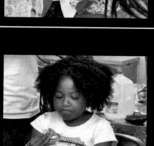

Electronics

Educational games and apps are another special-treat entertainment item in our house.

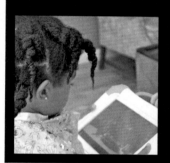

TV or Movies

My daughter's favorite activity is TV or movie time, which is reserved only for styling days.

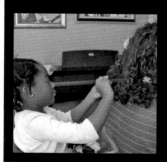

Family Hair

While doing your child's hair, let your child practice on another family member. It can be both fun *and* funny!

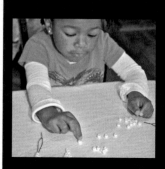

Counting

Putting some beads in the hairstyle? Have your child count them out into groups for you while you're styling.

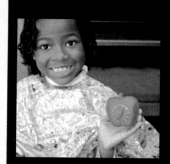

Using Timers

Having a timer or stop-watch available for your child to keep track of time before breaks gives her a sense of control.

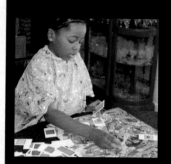

Board Games

If your child is concerned with being singled out, get everyone involved during styling with family game time.

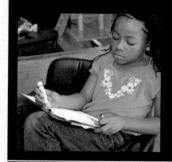

Drawing

Drawing during styling is all sorts of fun, especially when my daughter illustrates hairstyles she wants me to try.

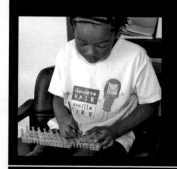

Elastic Loom

Not only a good distraction, this activity is a great use of the old elastics I used when my daughter was younger.

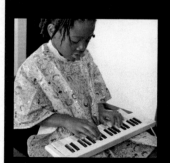

Music

Playing a musical instrument or singing with the family is another great way to enjoy hair time together.

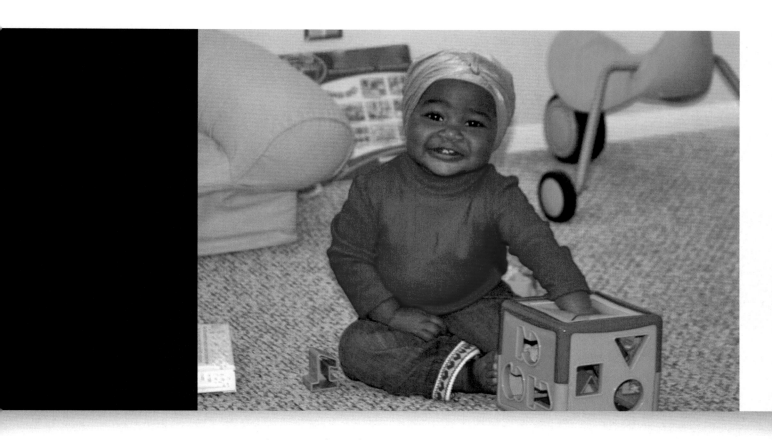

PART VI
HAIRSTYLE MAINTENANCE

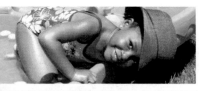

HOW TO PROTECT HAIRSTYLES

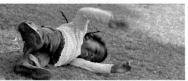

PLAYTIME

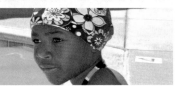

SWIMMING

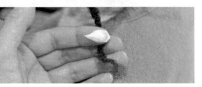

MAINTAINING STYLES

HOW TO PROTECT HAIRSTYLES

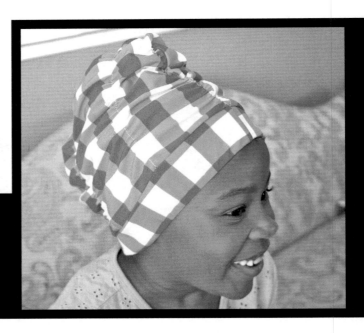

MURPHY'S LAW OF HAIR

Assume that immediately after you finish a hairstyle, something will happen to it to mess it all up.

So, you've invested time in learning how to do something special with your child's hair, and it doesn't look half-bad. Congratulations! Then your child has dinner and half of it ends up in her hair, or you pick her up from preschool with a head full of sand.

It's hard to watch your hard work unravel so quickly due to circumstances beyond your control. But for everyday maintenance, you and your child can certainly take some preventative steps to help preserve your hairstyling efforts.

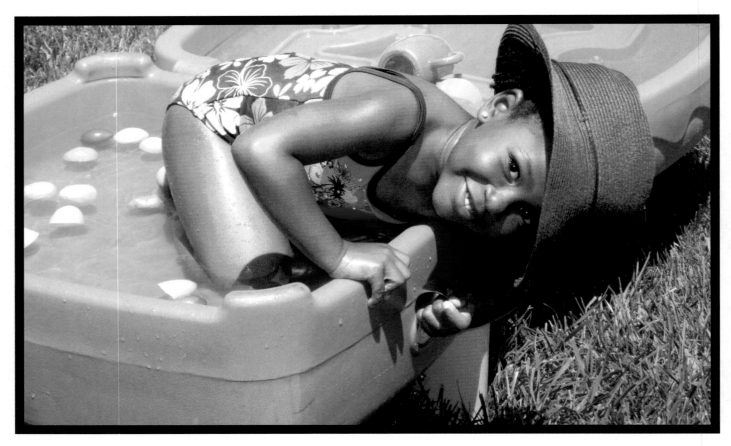

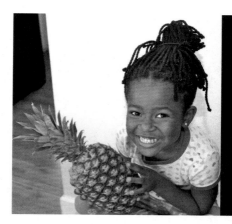

PINEAPPLING

Pineappling refers to gently gathering the hair up to the top of the head, like a pineapple. It is done to minimize friction on the ends of the hair while sleeping (preferably on a satin pillowcase or with a sleep cap). A terrycloth O and boxed hairstyles work best for this method.

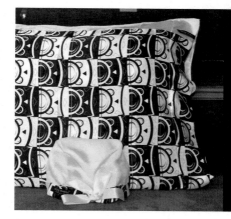

SATIN PILLOWCASES

A satin pillowcase is an excellent option for kids who, for one reason or another, cannot keep a sleep cap on at night. Satin does not draw moisture away from the hair like cotton does. Additionally, it provides slip between the hair and the pillow, a huge plus for active sleepers. Satin pillowcases are also a great option for boys who don't feel comfortable wearing a "do-rag."

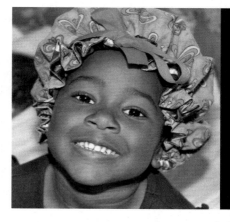

SLEEP CAPS

In our house, we use sleep caps in conjunction with satin pillowcases. The satin-on-satin slip between the two makes sleeping more comfortable for my daughter. In addition, sleep caps provide added protection by keeping the hair nicely bundled on top of the head where it is less likely to get caught on anything during the night. Lycra sleep caps also make a great option for protecting hair against sand at the beach.

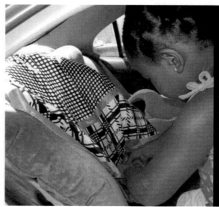

CAR SEATS

As a toddler, my daughter had no problem wearing a sleep cap while strapped in her car seat, especially during the daytime. Now that she's older, it's not something she feels comfortable doing. Instead, we've attached a satin scarf to the back of the car seat. In addition to providing slip and moisture protection, much like the satin pillowcase, the scarf also helps protect her car seat from hair product build-up.

PLAYTIME

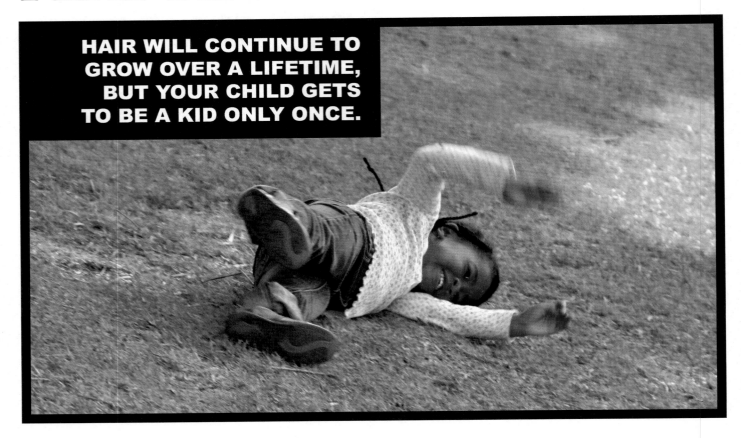

HAIR WILL CONTINUE TO GROW OVER A LIFETIME, BUT YOUR CHILD GETS TO BE A KID ONLY ONCE.

Kids are kids. They play. They roll in grass, get sweaty, play in mud, and stomp in puddles without a second thought. Hair is going to get tangled, it's going to snag on a tree branch when running too close, and sometimes it may even break. Your child may even enjoy the rite of passage that comes with trimming her hair, invariably in that one conspicuous spot in the front that just can't be hidden.

It's reasonable to want to protect the work you put into a hairstyle, but that protection should never come at the price of a child's ability to play like all of the other kids. The unique needs of natural hair (and the styles used to protect it), however, may require some clever work-arounds. On the following page, I've outlined some of my tips for coping with the things that happen when kids play like, well, kids.

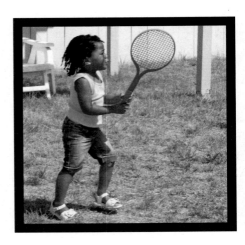
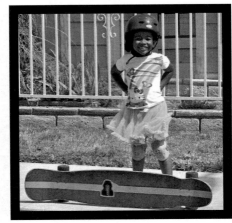
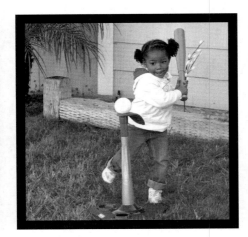

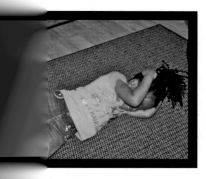

ROLLING AROUND

Doing somersaults, rolling down a grassy hill, or just plain rough housing on the floor can wreak havoc on a hairstyle. Picking out dust bunnies, leaves, and grass are pretty normal with little kids and is just a regular part of everyday hair maintenance. As they grow older, children will better understand the implications of certain types of activities on their hair and may choose to alter how they play because of it. How you respond to these instances will set the tone for how your child and your family approach playing with regards to hair.

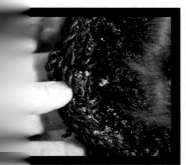

SAND & DIRT

For sandboxes and trips to the beach, my daughter and I use Lycra swim caps (or sleep caps) to help protect her hair. When her hair is unprotected, I remove sand and dirt by using either an air compressor (on low) to blow it out or a vacuum attachment (on low) to suck it out. Be sure that the hair is dry when doing this so that sand or dirt will loosen more quickly. Fungi (like ringworm) can live in sand and dirt, so be sure to wash the hair after removing the larger grains.

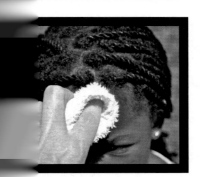

SWEAT

In addition to becoming a breeding ground for fungi and bacteria, sweat can also cause odor. A great way to combat sweat is to style the hair off the neck and shoulders. If the scalp does get sweaty, rinsing it with warm water is a great way to purge sweat and particles that were picked up during play. Be sure to remoisturize afterward. If a water rinse is not practical, wet a towel with warm water and gently wipe or dab the part lines and hairline *before* the sweat dries.

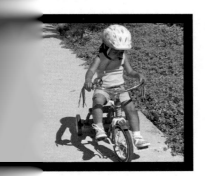

HELMETS

Many helmets often utilize pieces of foam attached by Velcro, which may snag hair. Even for helmets without Velcro, I like to place a thin satin or Lycra cap underneath the helmet to protect the hair from both friction and from the possibility of getting caught. Using a cap that matches your child's hair color draws little attention to the fact that she is wearing it. Or you can get one that matches the color of the helmet.

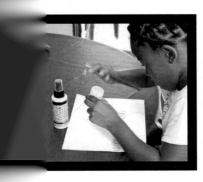

GLITTER

Glitter gets on the skin and in the hair and it's difficult to get out. I've found Christmas glitter in the hair several months after the holidays. It happens. When it does, I like to blow out as much of it as I can with an air compressor (on low) and then use a piece of transparent tape wrapped around my finger to dab at the rest. The tape is sticky enough to catch the glitter, but not so sticky that it breaks my daughter's hair. Be sure to test your child's hair strength first in order to avoid breakage.

SWIMMING

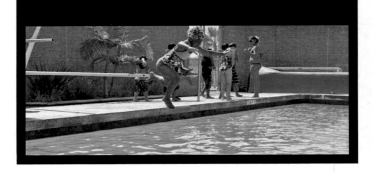

How to protect natural hair while swimming is probably the number one question parents ask during the summer months. Even for our straight-haired friends, swimming in the ocean or in chlorinated pools can damage hair. However, taking a few precautionary steps will allow your naturally curly child as much opportunity to enjoy swimming as the next child, while still maintaining a healthy head of hair.

Chlorine and salt both dry out hair because they strip away its natural oils, leaving the strands exposed to either chemicals or moisture loss. When the hair is devoid of its natural oils, it can become overly porous (*i.e.,* damaged). The more you swim, the more the protective oils are depleted, and the more vulnerable the hair strands become.

Have you ever wondered why blond hair sometimes turns green from swimming in chlorinated pools? That's what happens when hair absorbs oxidized metals, much like what happens to a penny when it oxidizes and turns green. The less protected the hair (*i.e.,* the more oils that are stripped away), the easier it is for those oxidized metals to penetrate the hair shaft. Green hair is a perfect example of just how harsh swimming can be on hair when it's not properly protected.

Although darker hair can also acquire a slightly greenish tint too, particularly under certain types of lighting, most of the time we really only notice the tangled, dried-out mess that results from hair that has been damaged. Either way, swimming can cause problems on all types of hair, and not just for curly-headed kids. In fact, the tips outlined on the following pages are applicable to anyone who swims regularly. As with most things related to natural hair, it will likely take some experimenting with the different options to figure out what works best for you and your family.

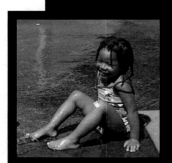

No Cap

With or without a cap, natural hair needs special care when swimming in order to keep it moisturized and prevent breakage.

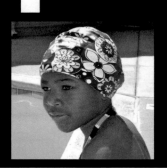

Silicone Caps

Water-resistant. Most frequently recommended for natural hair because they have a bit more slip to them and tend to pull less than latex caps.

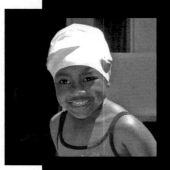

Latex Caps

Water-resistant. Latex caps are known to catch easily on hair. In addition, many people have latex allergies, so keep that in mind when shopping.

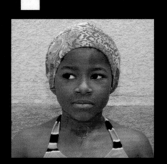

Lycra Caps

Non-water-resistant caps. Good for keeping the hair out of the face while swimming. Makes a good "undercap" for silicone or latex caps.

Swimming With a Swim Cap

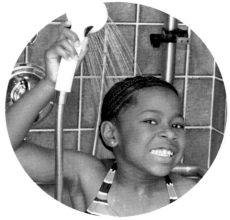
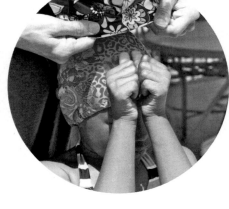

WET HAIR (optional)

Since no swim cap is entirely waterproof, we like to proactively neutralize any moisture that seeps into the cap by first wetting the hair with fresh water. If the hair is saturated with fresh water, it won't absorb any more moisture. Or, put another way, any chlorinated or salt water that makes its way into the cap won't penetrate the hair if it's already full of fresh water. This step is entirely optional, especially if you haven't had issues with water leaking into your child's swim cap.

LYCRA CAP (optional)

After saturating the hair with water, we like to put on a Lycra cap before adding a silicone cap. We do this for two reasons: First, it helps hold the hair in place, especially boxed hairstyles with lots of loose braids or twists; second, it provides an added layer of protection from any breakage that might happen when adding or removing the silicone (or latex) cap.

SWIM CAP

Putting on a swim cap is intuitive for older kids, but younger ones will likely need assistance. We use the method shown above, where my daughter will hook her two thumbs under the front of the cap, while an adult or friend helps her slip the cap over the rest of her head. Only when the cap is in its final place does she remove her thumbs, eliminating the slack that allowed the cap to be repositioned.

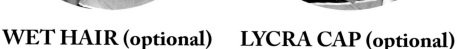

PROS	CONS
• Simply the best way to protect against the damaging effects of chlorine and salt by keeping the hair from becoming overly saturated with water or chemicals that strip its protective oils. The degree to which they will keep water of out the hair will vary; my daughter prefers to wear her caps over her ears, which helps the cap create a better seal.	• Putting on and taking off can snag or break hair. • Often requires two people to get them on and off. • May not fit over all hairstyles. • Can make a child feel self-conscious if she is the only kid wearing one. • Work best when covering the ears, which some kids may find uncomfortable.

Swimming Without a Swim Cap

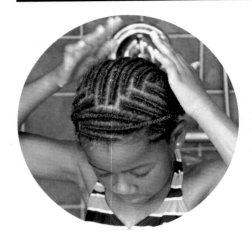

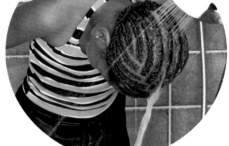

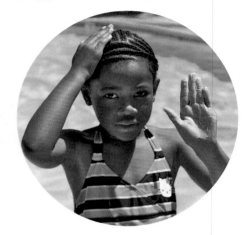

CONDITION

When going without a swim cap, we like to saturate the hair both with water and an inexpensive conditioner. Adding an extra layer of protection, the conditioner helps prevent the fresh water from evaporating, which would leave the hair exposed to an influx of chlorine or salt. You can either use a spray bottle to spray the conditioner, or rub it on your hands and pat it onto the head. Whether or not your child can do this on her own will depend on her age.

RINSE

After swimming, thoroughly rinse all of the water and conditioner out of the hair. Although this helps remove any unwanted pool or sea water, it will also deplete the hair of any moisturizing products, including the conditioner applied in the previous step. It's more important to make sure that the damaging water is removed, so don't worry about rinsing away products. The last thing you want to do is seal in damaging water when remoisturizing in the next step.

MOISTURIZE

Once the hair is thoroughly rinsed, it's time to add products. Some hairstyles are easier to remoisturize than others. For flat braids and twists, my daughter will pat a moisturizer into her hair, and then we will seal it with an oil and water spritz. For braids and twists, you can add moisture by smoothing it first into your hands and then squeezing it into each individual twist. Be sure to use a sealant if not already included in your moisturizing product.

PROS

- A child won't feel self-conscious about being the only one wearing a swim cap.
- Can be done with any hairstyle (although some more easily than others).

CONS

- Some pools will restrict hair product usage, including conditioners.
- Requires a lot of effort before and after swimming to ensure proper care.
- Constant manipulation of the hair can cause breakage.

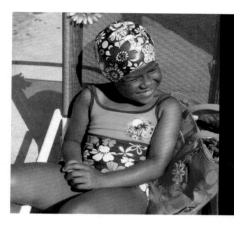

HAIRSTYLES FOR SWIMMING

Box braids and twists are usually the easiest for swimming without a cap as they can be easily rinsed and maintained, both before and after swimming. Cornrows and flat twists are excellent choices to wear under swim caps as they are usually flush to the scalp, allowing for a better fit. Extensions will work fine with or without swim caps; although making sure that you have the right sized cap for the extra hair is important, as is making sure that the extensions dry before they get smelly.

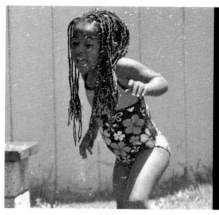

YARN EXTENSIONS

Be aware that yarn, when wet, will get very heavy and can pull on the hair. The extra weight of the saturated yarn can also cause the extensions to slip from their anchored point or break the hair, so use your discretion. Further, it takes a long time for yarn to dry; it can get a little musty-smelling if left wet for too long. If you want to use a swim cap with yarn extensions, I've found that using a Lycra cap first and then using an extra large, or long-haired, silicone cap on top works very well.

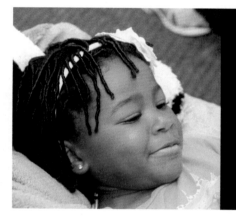

LOCS

Just like any other hairstyle, swimming with locs can be done with or without a swim cap. However, if locs are new or haven't been established for very long, it would be best to use a swim cap to make sure that they don't come out. As with longer hair and extensions, it's always helpful to band the hair on top of the head to make sure that the bulk of the hair goes into the area of the cap that has the most space and is off the hairline.

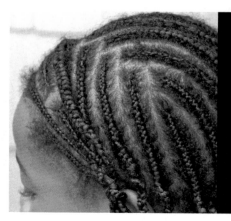

ADJUSTING HAIRSTYLE EXPECTATIONS

Regardless of whether or not you choose to use a swim cap, hairstyles simply do not remain crisp and fresh when swimming regularly. Friction from adding and removing caps, coupled with the constant swelling and shrinking that happens with repeated wetting and drying, will make even the most skillfully braided style pop with fuzzies. If the hair is well moisturized and not breaking, and the scalp is healthy, fuzzies and loose braids or twists are totally normal and are to be expected.

MAINTAINING STYLES

STYLE FOR MAINTENANCE

Some hairstyles fare better than others in certain circumstances. Weather conditions, children's activities, and sleep patterns all affect how long a style will last. It also helps to understand how much maintenance goes into the different types of protective styles to better determine which ones will best serve your family.

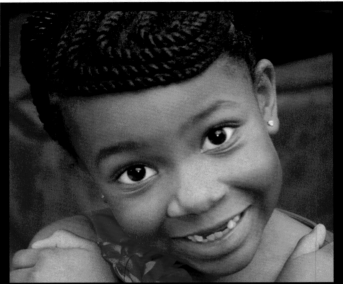

WEATHER

- For dry months, or months when it's cold and you're running the heater, add moisture back to the air by using a humidifier.
- Consider a thin satin cap under hats and caps to protect against friction and moisture loss.
- Be sure your child stays hydrated.
- For humid weather, reassess your use of products that contain humectants as they will cause the hair to absorb more water and frizz easier.

ACTIVITY

- Style off the neck and shoulders to combat sweat.
- Protect the hair from friction and moisture loss when wearing helmets and swim caps.
- Be sure to keep the scalp clean by addressing dirt, sand, and product build-up.
- Try to avoid pulling the hair up into ponytails too frequently as playtime can put extra tension on the edges.

SLEEP

- How often your child sleeps or naps will directly affect how long a hairstyle will last. The less sleeping, the less time spent rolling around on the hairstyle, especially if your child is an active sleeper.
- Use a satin pillowcase or a sleep cap.
- Remove all accessories before sleeping. Aside from being uncomfortable, they can also cause breakage by rubbing against the hair.

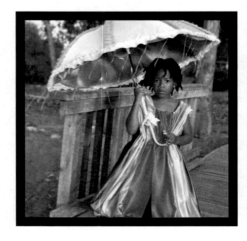

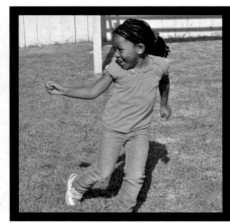

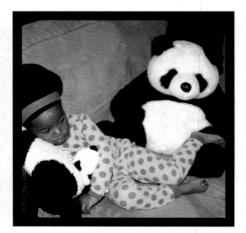

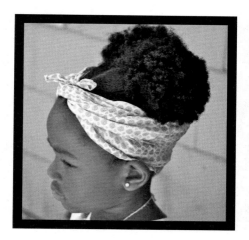

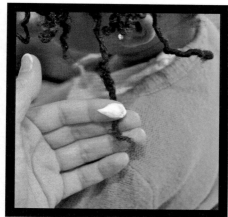

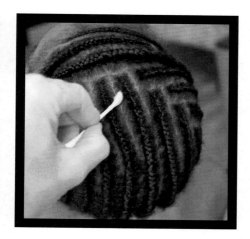

| BUNS & PUFFS | BOX BRAIDS & TWISTS | CORNROWS & FLAT TWISTS |

BUNS & PUFFS

- Check bun and redo as needed.
- Check edges for breakage. If breakage occurs, remove style.
- Check ends of puffs and moisturize as needed. Be sure to remove any items that may have found their way into the hair (*e.g.,* lint, grass, *etc.*).
- If the hair gathered into the puff or bun begins to get fuzzy, use either your hands (as I do) or a soft bristle brush to work in some gel or styling cream. Wrapping a scarf on top afterward helps keep the hairs in place while the product dries.

BOX BRAIDS & TWISTS

- Check the ends of all the boxes and add moisturizing cream as needed.
- If the braids or twists are sticking out, you can add clips to weigh down the ends and stretch them back into place.
- Spritzing with your favorite moisturizing mixture can help maintain moisture, but note that doing so will cause the hairstyle to become fuzzy quicker. Use your discretion.
- You can wash the hair with the style in.
- Rebraid or retwist any boxes that may be coming undone or need moisture.

CORNROWS & FLAT TWISTS

- Use a cotton swab and dab jojoba oil along the part lines to address dry patches on the scalp.
- If moisture is needed, spray with your favorite moisturizing spritz.
- Any itching or smell will indicate that the hair needs to be washed. Since washing will cause the hair to swell and increase fuzziness, use your discretion.
- Check for breakage and the health of the edges. Remove style if necessary.
- Address any moisture loss on the ends of braided or twisted rows as needed.

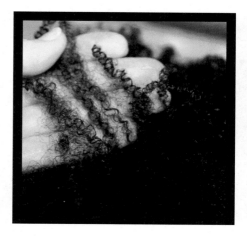

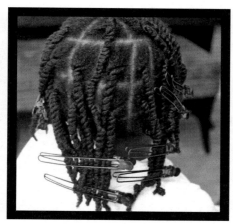

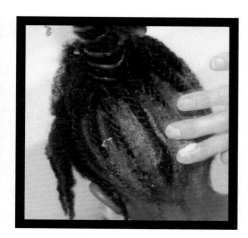

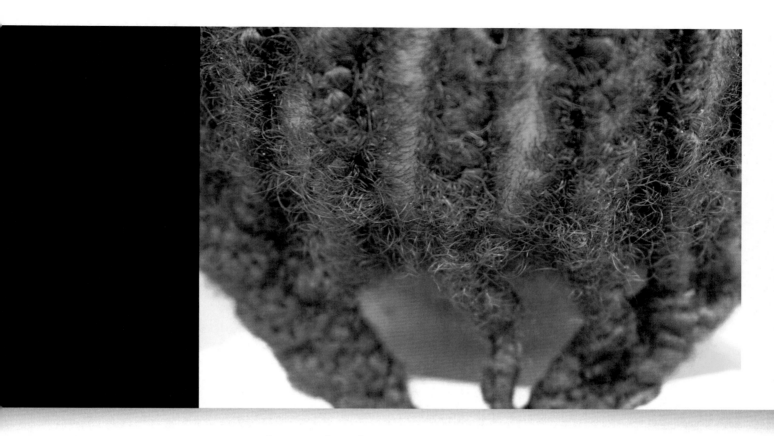

PART VII
REMOVING HAIRSTYLES

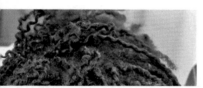

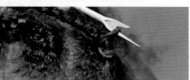

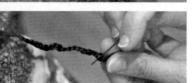

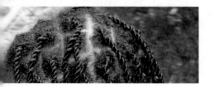

DECIDING WHEN TO RESTYLE

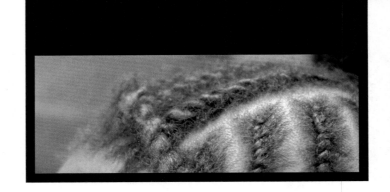

All hairstyles will get fuzzy at one point or another. Fuzzies are a fact of life in our house and boil down to a simple question of how many I'm willing to live with before I restyle. My general rule of thumb is that if I can still see the part lines, and none of the issues outlined on the following page are present, then the style is doing just fine. If fuzziness is something that bothers you, I've outlined some tips below on how to best minimize it.

Fuzziness does not necessarily mean a hairstyle needs to be removed. I've mentioned in earlier sections that humidity, spritzes, swimming, and activity can all play a role in generating fuzzies. However, careful attention does need to be paid for boxed hairstyles, especially in tightly coiled hair, as they can lock if left in for too long. I also recommend immediately removing a hairstyle for any of the reasons outlined on the following page.

MINIMIZING FUZZIES

Fuzzies happen when shorter lengths of hair pop out of the hairstyle. They happen on all hair types but are most noticeable with curly hair, because the popped ends curl up when freed, making them more visible.

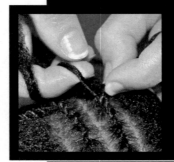

Styling

Styles that are pre-twisted last longer. Not exclusive to rope twists, you can also pre-twist the sections of braids to increase longevity.

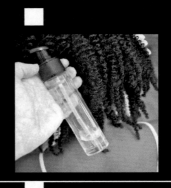

Products

Not properly sealing, or using the wrong types of products, can cause the hair to swell and shrink, thus popping out of the hairstyle.

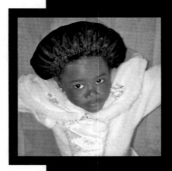

Friction

Spending less time rolling around on the hairstyle minimizes friction. Also consider styling off the shoulders and collars and avoiding pulling up into ponytails.

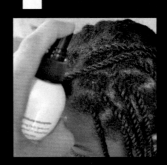

Care

Spraying water or moisturizers on the hair will cause it to swell, and then to shrink as it dries. Minimizing this process helps minimize fuzzies.

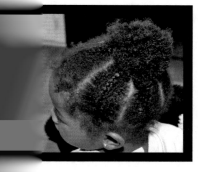

MOISTURE LOSS

A protective hairstyle is meant to protect the hair, specifically against moisture loss. If it's no longer doing what it's supposed to do, it's time to take it out. Many of today's natural hair products (if you're going the all-natural route) are water-based, so they will not hold moisture indefinitely. Even if you've sealed the hair well, time, friction, and evaporation will eventually chip away at that seal. You can usually see moisture loss most prominently along the edges of protective styles, or on the ends of boxed hairstyles.

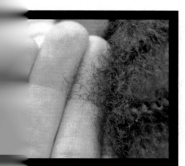

HAIR BREAKAGE

For many younger children, it is difficult to differentiate between fuzziness caused by breakage and fuzziness due to new hairs that have popped out of the style. You can tell if the hair is breaking if you see any strands in the sleep cap or on the pillow that *do not* have a little white bulb on the end; shed hair will *always* have the white bulb. Remove the style immediately if you're seeing broken hairs. Note that the longer you leave a style in, the more shed hairs you will notice when restyling; so don't panic.

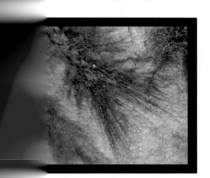

STRESSED SCALP

A "stress bump" on the scalp is a raised reddish area around the point where a strand of hair grows from the scalp. The redness and "bump" indicate too much tension is being placed on that strand of hair. They may or may not turn into white bumps (which can indicate clogged pores). Stress bumps are an early warning sign that the dermal papilla (the base of the hair follicle) is stressed; if the tension is not relieved, the dermal papilla and hair follicle can be permanently damaged, resulting in traction alopecia (*i.e.,* permanent hair loss).

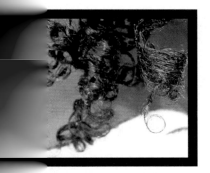

PRODUCT BUILD-UP

White flakes or flecks of dried product sitting *on top* of the hair (instead of having been *absorbed* into the strands) may indicate build-up. The scalp may also be a little flaky or you may find that the hair has an odor. Too much of any product, but especially one that is high in protein, can suffocate the hair, sealing out the moisture you're trying to add. Too much product in the hair can also facilitate matting and locking.

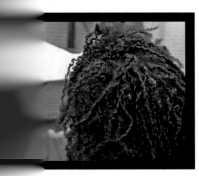

ODOR

If the hair smells at all, it's time to wash it. Some products will not mix well with others, and some items may not work with your child's body chemistry. Dirt, chlorine, food, or any number of other things that may have found their way into your child's hair during play, can all react and cause a smell. If the hair smells, something is not right. I highly recommend washing it immediately to avoid any possible infections or other complications.

Removing Elastics

TOOLS

- Seam ripper and/or
- Nail Clippers and/or
- Scissors

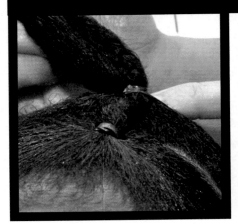
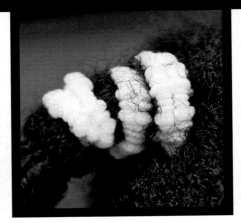
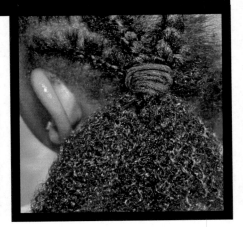

RUBBER BANDS

Never try to unwind or slip off rubber bands. They are made to be cut from the hair. That's why they're so cheap and sold in such large quantities. They are not intended for reuse, so don't feel badly about trashing them. This is assuming that the hair products have not already broken them. When it's time to remove them, my favorite go-to tool is a seam ripper. It can loop easily beneath the band and cut it without ever catching on the hair. I've also had great success with nail clippers when removing these tiny bands.

TERRYCLOTH O's

How you use terrycloth O's will best determine how you should remove them. If they're being used to stretch the curl pattern by banding the hair overnight (or even for a few days), then they will likely slip out with ease. If you've used them on the ends of boxed styles, they should slip right off. When using terrycloth O's at the base of boxes, especially for styles that have been in for a while, hair has probably managed to wrap around the band. At that point, it's best to use a pair of scissors to cut them out. Better safe than sorry.

PONY O's

If used to secure braids or twists, Pony O's can often be removed by just unwinding, depending on how tightly they were banded and how long the style has been in. The tighter they are, or the longer they have been in, the more likely it is that hair has wound around the Pony O. If so, the Pony O's will need to be cut. If used to secure puffs, then it is even more likely that the free hair will at some point become tangled within the Pony O, again requiring cutting. It is best to use a pair of scissors to cut the pony O's, especially when using the larger, thicker bands.

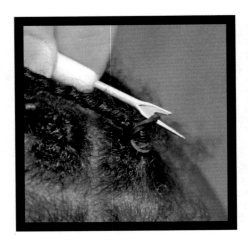
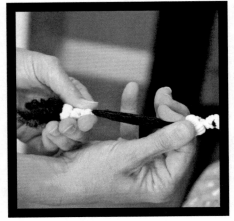
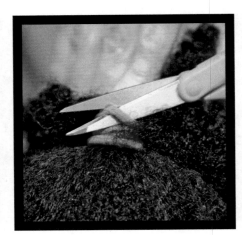

TOOLS

- Styling cream (to keep the ends from getting fuzzy while working)
- Spray bottle with water and lots of conditioner
- Either a darning needle or a pintail comb

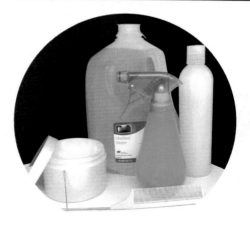

PREPARATION

In addition to the tools above, you will need a great deal of patience when removing tiny braids. Taking them out is an investment in hair health that should not be rushed.

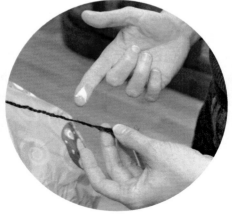

STEP 1

I like to spray the section of hair on which I'll be working with some water mixed with conditioner and let it soak in. I will then start with one braid and moisturize the ends to keep them from fuzzing up as I'm working.

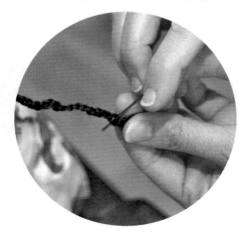

STEP 2

I prefer to use a darning needle to remove tiny braids. It's small and doesn't catch on the hair while I'm working. I also like not having to put it down when I want to use my fingers, as it tucks easily into my hand.

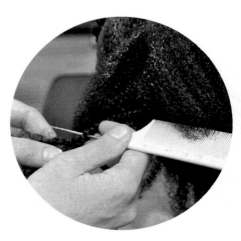

STEP 3

Others prefer to use a pintail comb, which also works great. Be sure to clip any hair out of the way, though, so that the comb will not catch on it while working.

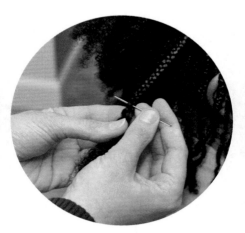

STEP 4

It is best to remove braids one stitch at a time. Trying to remove two or three stitches will likely cause the hair to tangle, so just go with one stitch until you get the hang of it.

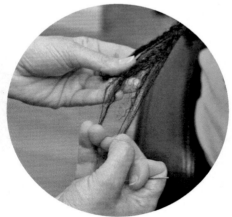

STEP 5

Once a stitch starts to separate, I like to let my fingers do the rest of the work. I can feel the tension on the hair better with my hands so I use my fingers whenever possible.

LOCKING & MATTING

For those who are unfamiliar, locked hair is simply a section of hair that is extremely tangled. In some contexts "locking" and "matting" are used interchangeably. Generally speaking, locking is often something that is done intentionally as a hairstyle, whereas matting is something that happens by accident.

All hair types can become matted. This is nothing specific to natural hair, although the curlier the hair is the more quickly it can happen.

Locs (the term used when referring to what most people know as "dreadlocks") are most likely to occur in boxed hairstyles, either intentionally or unintentionally (as happens sometimes). They usually begin locking at the base of the boxes, but can also start to tangle at the ends. Locking can happen for any number of reasons including leaving a style in for too long, product build-up, or excessive friction. Because tightly coiled hair can lock rather quickly, it's important to keep a close eye on hairstyles if this is something you're trying to avoid. For us, comb coils can lock in as little as a week; boxed braids and twists and can happen in about a month. How long it takes your child's hair to start locking will vary, so until you know with certainty how long you can keep in a specific style, pay careful attention to the possibility of it starting to lock.

If it happens, you can detangle it if you catch it early enough and have enough patience to do the job correctly. Remember that it's hair and, if worse comes to worse and there is some breakage, or if it needs to be cut, it will grow back.

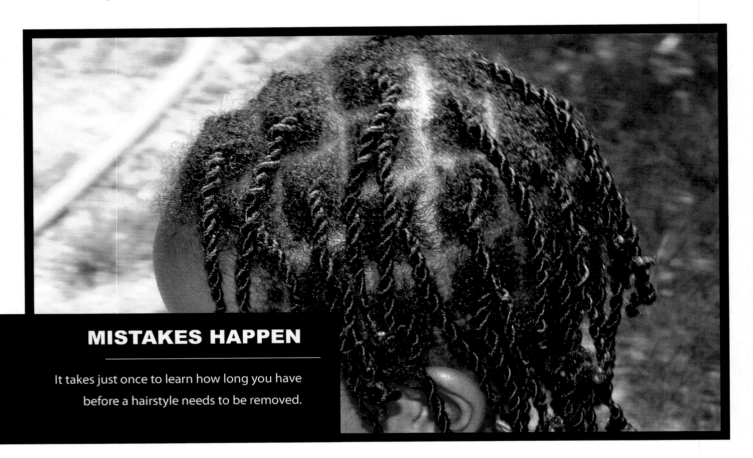

MISTAKES HAPPEN

It takes just once to learn how long you have before a hairstyle needs to be removed.

- Something that will break through grime and build-up (I like to use 2T apple cider vinegar in 8oz of water)
- A conditioner with tons of slip
- Ideally you want to exclusively use your fingers

Separating Tough Tangles

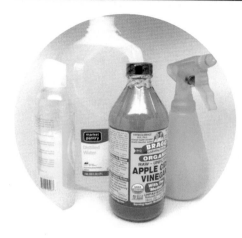

PREPARATION

Your fingers will be your most essential tool during this process. They will help you best determine how much tension the hair can handle as you work to lift and separate the hairs from one another.

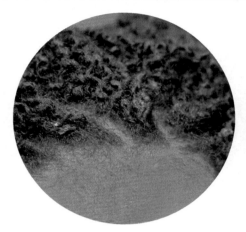

STEP 1

Start by using whatever product you've chosen to break through the grime and build-up in the hair. I usually spray with a mixture of distilled water and apple cider vinegar (ACV), letting it sit for a bit to work.

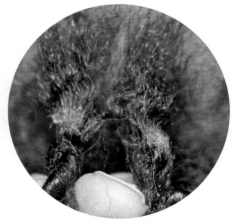

STEP 2

Once the build-up starts to loosen, I will move through the sections of hair with my fingers, gently separating the hair in the parts where the gunk is located, and picking out what I can while working the ACV in further.

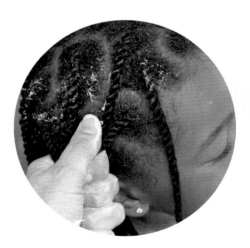

STEP 3

When I know the build-up is starting to break down, I will slather the tangled sections with a conditioner with lots of slip. I then allow the conditioner to sit for a bit and soak into the hair.

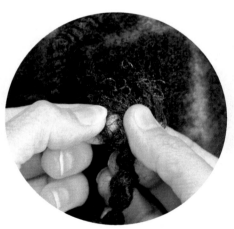

STEP 4

Work with one section at a time, slowly separating with your fingers. Once you've detangled a section, plait or twist it to keep it detangled and out of your way before moving on to the next section.

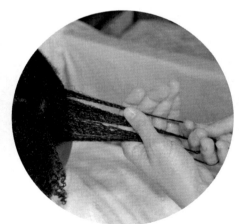

STEP 5

Go slowly, keeping the hair saturated with conditioner and water while working. Continue finger detangling until all stubborn tangles and gunk are removed. Then wash and detangle as normal.

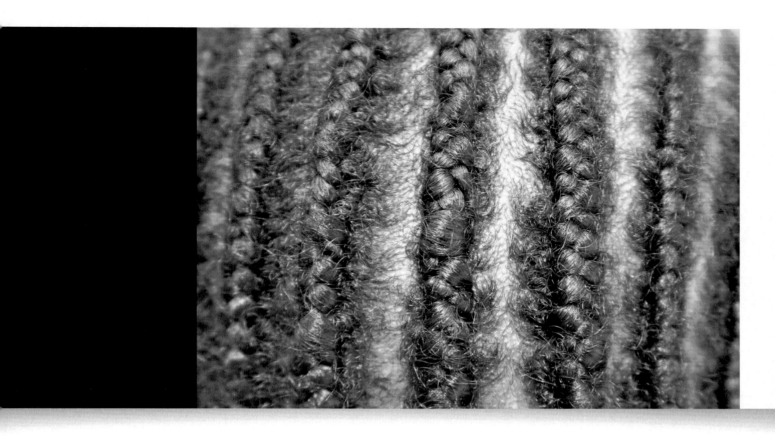

PART VIII
TROUBLESHOOTING

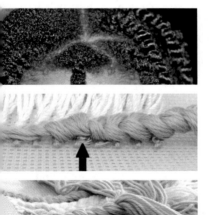

ISSUES WITH BOXED STYLES

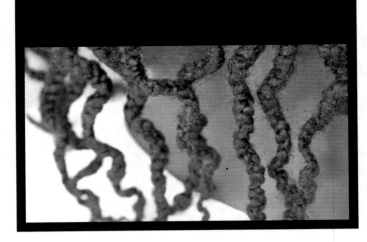

Several of the issues common to boxed styles have already been addressed in previous sections, such as how to straighten them if they're sticking out (use clips to weigh them down) and how to minimize fuzzies. I also wrote about how boxed styles can lock fairly quickly in some types of hair. Be sure to keep an eye on them and remove the style should you see any evidence of locking or matting.

For the most part, boxed hairstyles are pretty low-maintenance. The great thing about them is that if a coil, braid, or twist comes undone, gets something in it, or appears to be locking, you can easily address that single box without having to undo the entire style. Addressing individual boxes on an as-needed basis can increase the longevity of the hairstyle as well as reduce manipulation. Boxed braids and smaller boxed twists can also be cleansed with the style in if necessary.

The most common styling issue related to boxed styles is addressing boxes that have come undone or have started to unravel. I've outlined my solutions below.

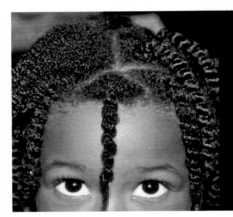

COMING UNDONE AT THE BASE

One of the biggest complaints about boxed styles (especially twists) is that they start to unravel or get puffy at the base. Technique helps, but it only goes so far. Using humectants in humid weather will cause the hair to puff with moisture, so a product change during those times may be in order. If the problem is not weather-related, you can band the hair at the base of the twist. Lastly, I suggest braiding a stitch or two at the base of a twist, which will draw the hair closer to the scalp.

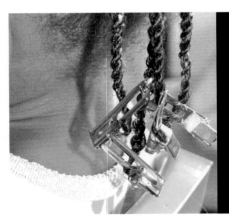

COMING UNDONE AT THE ENDS

As with braids and twists coming undone at the base, the ends can be held in place with bands. However, many times you can just clip the ends of your boxes until the hair dries. That way the hair will shrink and hold in the shape of the twist or braid, giving the product a chance to set. Once the hair is dry it is less likely to come undone. Braids usually hold better in hair that is not as tightly coiled, so doing a stitch or two of braids at the end of a twist can also help keep it in place.

Cornrows

A rolled cornrow (or braid) is something that happens when you accidentally braid in the same direction twice, causing the braid to twist. For example, instead of braiding right-under-center then left-under-center, you braid right-under-center twice, rotating the braid or cornrow.

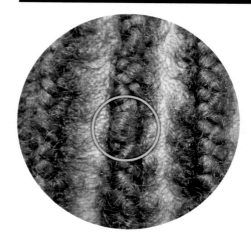

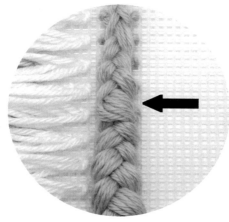

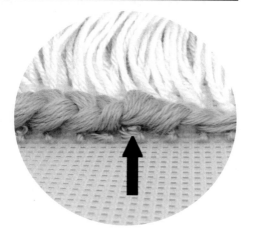

PROBLEM

You can identify where the cornrow has rolled when you see the presence of a "knot" that has broken the otherwise nicely-braided row of stitches.

EXPLANATION

When braiding cornrows, you must always alternate which side you're passing under the middle section. Passing the same side twice will roll the braid.

CLOSER LOOK

Depending on how tightly you braid, you may not actually roll the cornrow entirely or see a knot. But if there is a break in the pattern, this is usually the reason.

THE SOLUTION

The easiest way to fix rolled cornrows is to undo your stitches until you reach the knot. Back up one stitch before the break in the braid pattern to ascertain which side you had passed beneath your middle section. If you passed the right section, continue braiding with your next stitch going left-under-center. Continue braiding, making sure that you are alternating which side you're passing under the middle stitch in order to avoid rolling again. If you're new to braiding cornrows, it's easy to get distracted and forget which direction you passed on the previous stitch. It's okay to stop and back up a step to ensure you're making the correct choice; catching knots early prevents having to undo a row to fix them.

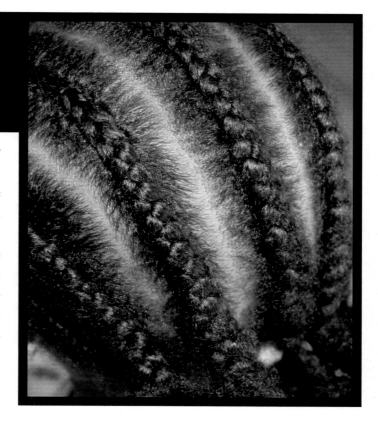

Tight Rows

Rows braided or twisted too tightly will often show puckering of the skin and could lead to permanent damage. Tight rows are most common to children with thinner or finer hair, as parents tend to overcompensate for hairs popping out by increasing tension.

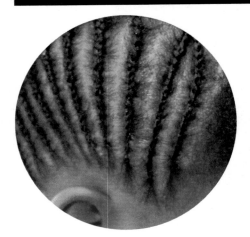

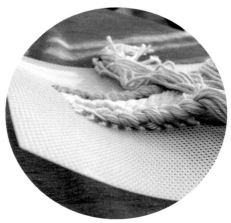

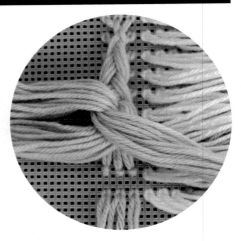

PROBLEM

The above rows were braided specifically to illustrate what the puckering of skin looks like when rows are too tight. You never want to see this on *any* hairstyle.

EXPLANATION

In the photo above, the hair being added to the braid is pulled upward into the row. As you can see, the tension causes the practice board to arc. Now imagine that tension on the scalp.

CLOSER LOOK

You can see the distance between the center section and the next row that needs to be pulled up into the stitch. Too much tension is required to secure the hair into the braid.

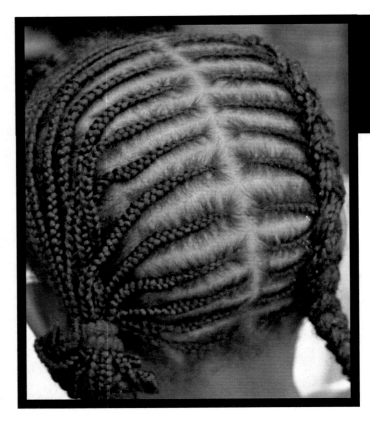

THE SOLUTION

To solve this problem, try skipping stitches so that the braid or twist remains positioned directly over the location of the new hair being added. Tutorials for skipping stitches are outlined on the following pages.

Sometimes people braid tightly on purpose in order to increase the longevity of the hairstyle. Braiding tightly is not the only way to achieve a smooth, crisp look. Let your hair products do the bulk of the work for you; use something with good hold so that you do not have to pull as tightly. In addition, try pre-twisting each section as you braid the row. It may take a little longer, but it will greatly minimize tension on the scalp and the results will last.

Skipping Cornrow Stitches

Skipping stitches is a way to ensure that your cornrows are not braided too tightly. The instructions below illustrate how to skip ONE STITCH, or put differently, how to add hair to EVERY OTHER STITCH of a cornrow. Skipping stitches is a great way to create evenly-spaced braids that are not too tight, especially for children with thinner or finer hair.

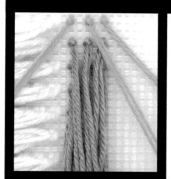

Part one row into three sections.

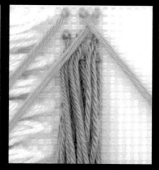

Swap right section under center.

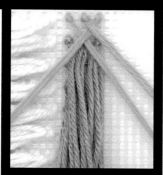

Swap left section under center.

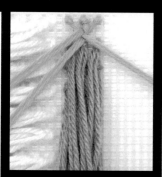

Swap right section under center.

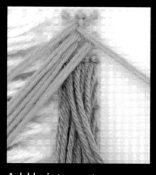

Add hair to center section.

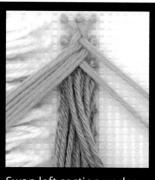

Swap left section under center.

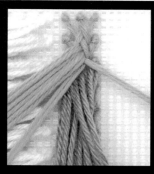

SKIP adding hair. Swap right section.

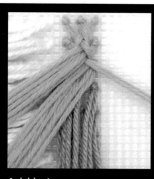

Add hair to center section.

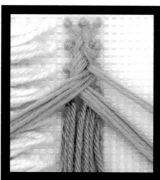

Swap left section under center.

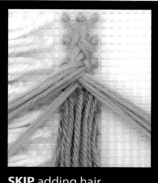

SKIP adding hair. Swap right section.

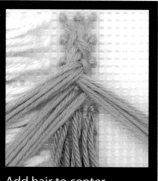

Add hair to center section.

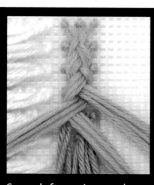

Swap left section under center.

A Parent's Guide to
Beginning Natural Hair Styling

Skipping Flat Twist Stitches

Skipping stitches is a way to ensure that your flat twists are not twisted too tightly. The instructions below illustrate how to skip TWO STITCHES, or put differently, how to add hair to EVERY THIRD STITCH of a flat twist. Skipping stitches is a great way to create evenly-spaced flat twists that are not too tight, especially for children with thinner or finer hair.

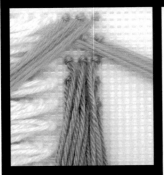
Start your twist with two sections.

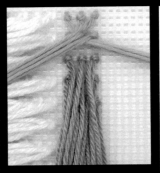
Swap the two sections, right over left.

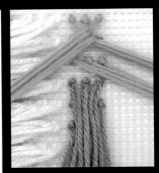
Add hair to the new right section.

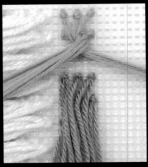
Swap the two sections, right over left.

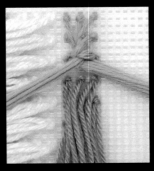
SKIP adding hair. Swap right over left.

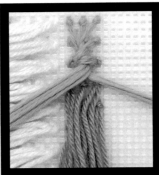
SKIP adding hair. Swap right over left.

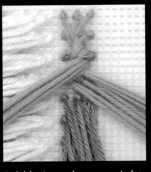
Add hair to the new right section.

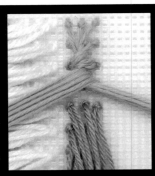
Swap the two sections, right over left.

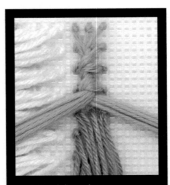
SKIP adding hair. Swap right over left.

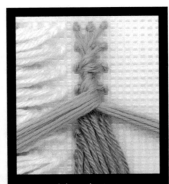
SKIP adding hair. Swap right over left.

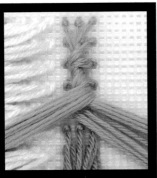
Add hair to the new right section.

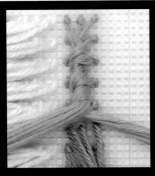
Swap the two sections, right over left.

Loose braids and twists do not have enough tension to keep the bottom portion close to the scalp. Whereas in tight rows the hair is being pulled upward into the braid, the hair being added in this case must be elongated downward to reach the braid or twist. Loose rows are most common to children with thicker or coarse hair.

Rows

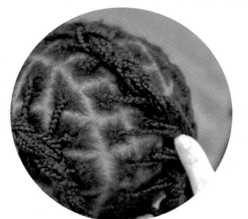

PROBLEM

The longer the row continues, the further away loose rows will float from the scalp. This is not necessarily bad, but the hair is more likely to slip out of the style when loose.

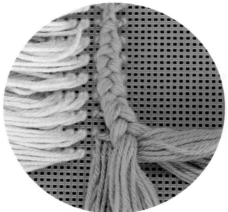

EXPLANATION

You can see above how the bottom portion of the braid can be moved to the side. This is a good technique for braiding rounded edges, but not the most protective.

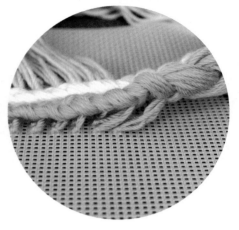

CLOSER LOOK

The photo above illustrates how the braid moves past the section of hair that gets added to it, so that the added hair becomes increasingly longer with each stitch.

THE SOLUTION

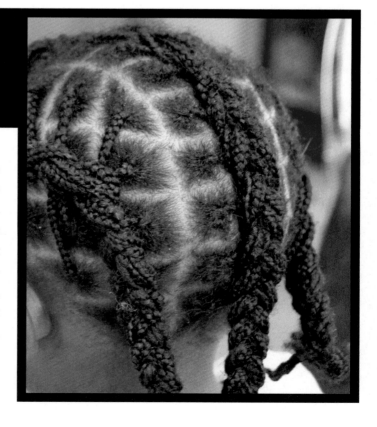

This is essentially the opposite problem of tight rows. In this case, your braid is getting *ahead* of the hair. The best way to solve this problem is to undo the row up to where it starts to move away from the scalp, and then add less hair into each of the stitches. If your cornrows or flat twists are consistently loose, you do not want to be skipping *any* stitches. In fact, you should be doing *more* stitches, adding smaller sections of hair with each stitch so that your cornrow or flat twist doesn't get too long before it's time to add more hair. This method should help keep your stitches in the same location as each new section of hair that you're adding, reducing the slack and making your rows more consistent in tension.

APPENDIX A
Sample Styling Routines

ROUTINE 1
BABY HAIR

CLEANSE

- Rinse with warm water at bath time. Bathing does not need to happen every day and can dry out the skin (and hair) if done more often than necessary.
- Wash with a conditioner or a sulfate-free shampoo only when absolutely necessary.

DETANGLE

- After cleansing.
- Use a light-weight (liquid) or spray leave-in conditioner.
- Detangle exclusively with your fingers.

MINIMIZE STYLING

- Delay styling your baby or toddler's hair until it becomes necessary to keep it moisturized and detangled.
- Avoid pulling on the hairline or tugging the hair into hairstyles.
- Pay careful attention to the use of accessories as they can be choking hazards for young children.

TYPES OF STYLES

- Finger coils are a great first hairstyle.
- When the hair is long enough, box twists and braids are recommended (preferably without the use of elastics).
- Try to avoid flat braids and twists until the child is older; babies and toddlers have tender scalps.
- Baby hair changes rapidly during the first few years, so it may not style in a predictable way until it reaches its final texture. Knowing this can help ease frustration as you're learning to style.

ROUTINE 2
KEEPING HAIR SHORT

CLEANSE

- Wash hair using a rinse-out conditioner (co-wash) every 3-7 days, as needed.
- Add a clarifying wash (a shampoo) if dirt or sweat is a factor. Also add a shampoo wash for older kids as they reach puberty. Follow a shampoo wash with a rinse-out conditioner.

DETANGLE

- If hair is long enough, use a leave-in liquid or spray conditioner with slip.
- Detangle exclusively with your fingers. If finger detangling is not enough, the hair may be too long to follow the short-hair styling routine.

MOISTURIZE

- Layer a creamy moisturizer after detangling for coarse or especially dry hair.
- For very short hair, this step will not be needed.

SEAL

- Layer a sealing oil or butter on top of the conditioner; also add after moisturizing, if not already included in the moisturizer.

MAINTAIN SCALP

- If hair is cropped close to the scalp, be sure to keep it moisturized. I recommend jojoba oil for scalp moisture, as it most closely matches sebum (natural scalp oil).

TRIM OR CUT THE HAIR REGULARLY

- Be sure to stay on top of hair cuts and trims. The longer the hair gets, the more likely you will need to style it, so if it's getting particularly dry or tangled, it's either time to change the hairstyle routine or get it cut.

ROUTINE 3
GROWING LONG HAIR

REMOVE PREVIOUS HAIRSTYLE

- Plait the hair into sections as you're removing the style to keep it detangled.

CLEANSE

- Wash hair weekly, in sections (see above).
- Use a rinse-out conditioner (co-wash). If styled to last longer than a week, co-wash with the style in as needed.
- Add a clarifying wash (a shampoo) if dirt or sweat is a factor. Also add a shampoo wash for older kids as they reach puberty. Follow a shampoo wash with a rinse-out conditioner.
- Add a chelating shampoo at least once a month for swimmers.

DEEP CONDITION

- Chemically processed hair should be deep conditioned weekly. Add a protein deep condition once a month.
- Swimmers or those with very dry or very long hair should also deep condition as needed.

DETANGLE

- Use a leave-in liquid conditioner with slip.
- Finger detangle as much as possible, following with a wide-toothed comb if necessary.

MOISTURIZE

- Layer a creamy moisturizer after detangling for coarse or dry hair.

SEAL

- Layer a sealing oil or butter on top of the conditioner; also add after moisturizing, if not already included in the moisturizer.

STYLE

- Style according to skill level, family needs, and hair goals.

Sample Styling Routines (continued)

Styling routines are not one-size-fits-all. With that in mind, I've outlined a few questions you may want to address as you and your child work together to discover what routine fits best with your family.

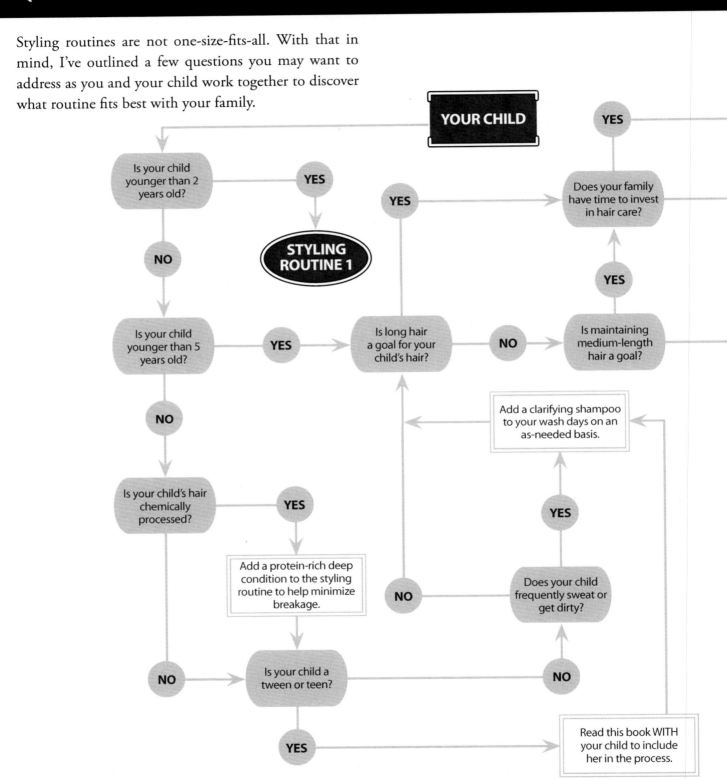

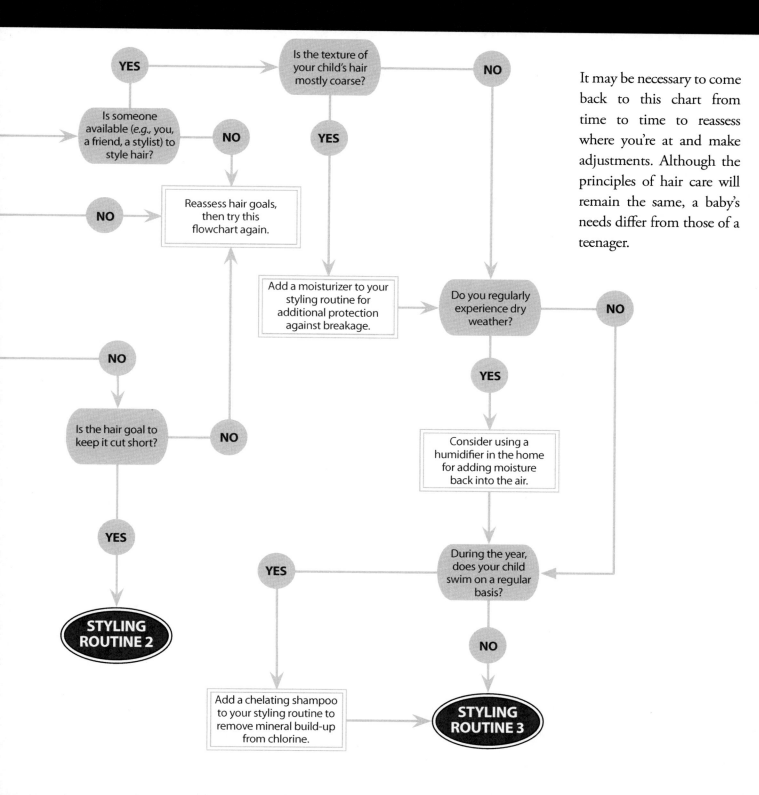

It may be necessary to come back to this chart from time to time to reassess where you're at and make adjustments. Although the principles of hair care will remain the same, a baby's needs differ from those of a teenager.

APPENDIX B
Hair Products

No hair product in the world is going to replace proper hair maintenance. The longer natural hair gets, the easier it tangles and the more quickly it loses moisture. The styling instructions outlined in this book are meant to help whichever hair products you choose to work better. If you are not taking these steps to ensure healthy hair maintenance, no product you buy will make up for that. Growing long curls takes work, and the longer they get, the greater the time investment required for their care. It is essential to keep this in mind when choosing products, as well as when determining hair goals. The hair care routine required for longer natural hair maintenance is not for everyone, nor will it fit the lifestyle of every family ... and that's okay! Understanding that natural hair is styled for reasons beyond culture and aesthetics is the first step in determining a natural hair routine that's right for your child.

DEFINING PRODUCT TYPES

Companies come and go and ingredients change faster than printed material. Furthermore, there is no standard when it comes to product labeling; what one company calls a moisturizer, another may call a conditioner. Therefore, I've defined my use of these terms in order to help you better assess products when shopping.

CONDITIONER

When conditioner is referenced as a product used in a style, I am referring to a leave-in conditioner or detangler, not the stuff that you rinse out after a wash. When layering products for a hairstyle, I'm only speaking of the products that will remain in the hair for the duration of the hairstyle. Whatever product you use for slip and conditioning during the detangling process, this is the "conditioner" to which I am referring.

MOISTURIZER

A moisturizer is not necessary for younger babies, some toddlers, or any child who has thin or finely textured hair. Moisturizers are heavier than detangling leave-in conditioners and can weigh hair down if not needed. This could make the hair limp, dull, and unnecessarily oily-looking. The moisturizers I'm referring to are water-based and are thick enough so that they won't run off your hand as a leave-in conditioner will.

SEALANT

Not usually included in leave-in conditioners, a sealant is absolutely necessary if you're only using a detangler as your moisturizer. For finer hair, a watered-down moisturizer makes a reasonable sealant. Thicker or more coarse hair will benefit from a carrier oil (like olive oil, castor oil, jojoba oil, or argan oil) or a butter (like shea butter, mango butter, or coconut oil) if not already included in the moisturizing product.

STYLING PRODUCT

Styling gels and creams are not intended to moisturize the hair. They are almost exclusively used for hold, so they are layered onto the hair *after* it has been moisturized and sealed. Not usually necessary for thinner, finer hair, a styling product should be free of drying ingredients (like petroleum and non-"fatty" alcohols) and applied only as needed to prevent build-up. Too much styling product can seal out moisture, so less is more.

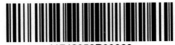

41742052R00060